HEALTH INSURANCE

Understanding it, and Medicare

Wayne Lackner

Published by:
Fee Publishing Co.
P.O. Box 681 H
Kent, Ohio 44240-0681

First edition. First printing.

Printed and bound in the United States

Library of Congress Catalogue #91-72257

Publisher's Cataloging-in-Publication Data:

   Lackner, Wayne C., 1944 -
      Health insurance : understanding it,
         and Medicare
            p. 153
         Includes bibliographical references, index.
         1. Insurance, health -- United States I. Title

   HG9396.L3   1992

   368.382'00973 -- dc 20

   ISBN 0-9629538-0-6

TABLE OF CONTENTS

Foreword & Introduction *I*

**Chapter 1 - A Little History
    (Understanding It, By Evolution)** *1*
      Major Medical *5*
      Historical Review *13*

Chapter 2 - Using Your Health Insurance *14*
      Review and Examples *22*
      Pre-Certification/Pre-Admission
      Cost Containment & Utilization Review *27*

Chapter 3 - Choosing Your Health Insurance *31*
      Prescriptions *34*
      In Conclusion and COBRA *36*

Chapter 4 - Buying Health Insurance
      The Deductible *39*

Chapter 5 - Exclusionary Riders, and Agents *48*
      Whom to Buy From *51*

Chapter 6 - Why Individual, and Why Not? *53*
      (Including Pre-existing Conditions)

Chapter 7 - Is it Cancellable? Or Re-Enterable? *63*

Chapter 8 - From Medicare to Medicaid *69*
    (Supplements and Long Term Care)
      Medicare – Part A *71*

Assignment and Appeal *74*
Part B *77*
Exclusions *79*
Medicare Supplements
    (Medigap) Coverage *81*
Nursing Home Policies
    (Long Term Care) *85*
Medicaid *91*

Chapter 9 - Trends, Taxes and Trivia *93*
Federal Taxes *99*
State Taxes *101*
Trivia *103*

Chapter 10 - Dental, Disability, Etc... *109*
Disability Income *112*
Dreaded Disease Coverage *115*
Extra Trivia *117*

Appendix - Odds and Ends
Surgery Requiring A Second Opinion *119*
Questionable Surgery *120*
General Exclusions *124*
Partially Covered Expenses *125*
Height and Weight Charts *128*
Declinations *132*
Suggestions *137*

Glossary of Special Terms *139*

Suggested Reading (Bibliography) *147*

Index *151*

Foreword &
Introduction

This book is written to be informational; but, in a conversational tone. My purpose is to help you understand health insurance in a kind of philosophical way (that is, how *it* works). The book is based on my experiences selling health insurance, and is a guide to how things really are out there in the world. Most of what I have learned has been gained from listening to other people talk about their problems and experiences–some to whom I've sold policies, and some who have just sold me.

As I was writing the book, I was reminded of the many presentations that I had made with Ma and Pa, the kids, and the dog (nibbling on my pants legs) at the kitchen table. I guess that I'm trying to invite myself into your home, so that I can tell you my story. I have tried to make the story flow as smoothly as possible; but, unfortunately, the facts kept getting in the way. I have tried to deal with them without losing the point.

Most of all, it is my sincere desire (along with selling books) that by reading this book, you will benefit from it–much more than what you invest in time or money–in which case it will be a win/win relationship. I have learned an awful lot about health insurance since I started. I hope that you will, too.

After my career of traveling (several years was enough to make me weary), I developed my own local agency as an agent/broker dealing with small-medium-sized businesses and employers. From this experience, I gained an insight into the problems that employees have using and choosing their health insurance. It also forced me to get involved with the claims-handling end of the business. I was as reluctant as anyone; but, like riding a bicycle, it wasn't as hard as I had anticipated–and there is a compensating reward: once you learn it this way, you will always remember.

Most people that work at insurance companies, even underwriters, are human beings; and dealing with them, even long-distance (the better companies have toll-free numbers) isn't as difficult as you might imagine. There is also the satisfaction that justice is usually served, although the process may seem slow at times. If you do your part, in most cases, they are willing to do theirs. Sometimes an effort is necessary that seems unfair–usually because of miscommunication–but, like learning about something, it's worth it in the end.

By the way, if you skip around the book, it's OK. For specific information use the index; but, you might miss the general understanding of the subject, if you don't read it through. Even if you are only interested in Medicare, you should read the beginning and early chapters about Blue Cross/Shield, first. Also, reading about Medicare, after the other chapters, will help you understand health insurance, in general. They are all related, and when you see them together in the same light, you will know what I mean.

Wayne Lackner – Kent

CHAPTER 1 – A LITTLE HISTORY
(UNDERSTANDING IT, BY EVOLUTION)

Why do we have health insurance, in fact, why do we have insurance, at all? Modern insurance began as a pooling of risk -- probably the best example would be Lloyd's of London who has insured merchant ships crossing the seas throughout the British Empire, around the world, since 1688. Basically, the shipowner paid a premium (or percentage) of the ship's value and cargo to the House of Lloyd's, who determined the risk factor at the time. If the ship didn't return in a certain period of days, months, or years, then the shipowner would be reimbursed the face value that had been issued on the policy. This was (is) called "casualty" insurance which now includes cars, homes, businesses, etc.

Life insurance was another development of English logic and ingenuity. In America, the first corporation with a life insurance purpose was organized in 1759, and was known as the "Presbyterian Ministers' Fund". The ministers paid an annual premium during their lifetimes, to provide an income for their widows and children. This was more than an annuity because it guaranteed a widow's income for her lifetime and the children's incomes for 13 years after the father's death[1].

Accident insurance was the next development toward health insurance. It sounds like a casualty-type risk; but, it is underwritten by life insurers. Basically, accident insurance covers bodily harm due to an accidental injury. Most of these policies would indemnify the policy owner, or pay a pre-determined amount for a specific injury. Example: $500 for accidental loss of limb, or sight in one eye; $1,000 for loss of two limbs, etc. This type of coverage was eventually incorporated into life insurance policies, especially group plans, later on.

Now, health insurance, as we know it (the kind that is sold by life insurance companies) evolved from the accident policies when coverage for sickness was added. Very few of these policies were sold early-on because most people had Blue Cross to cover hospital expenses. Actually, early in this century most people didn't have any health coverage, and few had life insurance. They either didn't have the money to pay premiums or the reason to have insurance.

The need for insurance is created when something has, or is perceived as having, value. A hundred years ago, the average man didn't care about buying life insurance, especially when *he* had to *die* for anyone to benefit from it. Also, families were closer and more willing to care for each other. In fact, you didn't even need burial insurance, because they would show you in the parlor, and then cart you off to the churchyard.

The biggest impetus to the widespreading of health insurance was the establishment of Blue Cross. In 1929, a group of schoolteachers (in Dallas, Texas) thought it would be a good idea to give the local hospital fifty cents a month (in advance) so that when it came time for them to have their babies, they could go there, and they wouldn't owe a bill.[2] This was basically a premium paid to the hospital; but, it was different than insurance in that it was really a pre-payment plan for expected service. The ones that signed up for it and didn't have babies were most likely unhappy; but, they probably didn't ask for a refund either. From a maternity plan it was an easy step to a hospital plan that would cover sicknesses and accidents and what we call "hospitalization" (or Blue *Cross*).

Blue *Shield* was the next step in the evolution: As doctors got more expensive, the logical thing was to include them, for a few

3

dollars more a month. The first such medical-surgical plan was developed in 1939, and called the "California Physicians' Service".[3] From fifty cents a month to have babies in the hospital, we are now paying a few hundred dollars a month (family coverage) for a variety of services.

About 30 years ago (in the early 1960's) most of the people who had decent health coverage, had Blue Cross which is not actually insurance; but, as noted, is a prepayment plan. Kaiser Permanente, as a pioneer in the health maintenance organization (H.M.O.) business, had some (mostly in California), and then there were some who had "sickness and accident" policies, from life insurance companies (indemnity policies, aside).

About 20 years ago (in the 1970's) the Blues (which includes Blue Cross, Blue Shield and major medical) began to get expensive, and attractive (premium-wise) to the life insurers. When the Blues went over $200 a month for family coverage (in the midwest) which was $300 or more on the coasts (San Francisco, Los Angeles, New York, Philadelphia, Chicago, Cleveland, etc.), the life insurers started to get more into the market. The policies that emerged were an interesting variety of improved "sickness and accident" policies, copies of basic Blue Cross/Blue Shield and some new "major medical" plans.

MAJOR MEDICAL

Major medical is one of the most confusing terms in health coverage – it doesn't mean exactly what it sounds like. The best way to understand it, is to explain how it has evolved.

First, there was Blue Cross, which pays the hospital, then there was Blue Shield, which pays the doctor in the hospital (ancillary services, assistant surgeons and technicians which have evolved since basic coverage began are split up between Blue Cross and Blue Shield depending on whether they are hospital or medical-surgical costs).

Then, in the 1950's, when we had to have it all, major medical expense coverage evolved on the scene. In 1949, Liberty Mutual introduced major medical expense benefits to supplement basic hospital and medical-surgical expenses.[4] In other words, major medical was to be a catch-all for expenses that exceeded the basic coverage (Blue Cross and Blue Shield). So, it included doctor visits (at the office), prescriptions, crutches and other medical care expenses. Well, it didn't take too long before everybody was visiting the doctor, taking prescriptions, and incurring other, extra expenses to such a degree, that a discouragement had to be invented.

If you didn't guess, the deductible had arrived. In most cases, in the beginning, deductibles on major medical expenses were around $100. Along with the deductible, came co-insurance. Usually, and until recently, the co-insurance was paid 80% by the plan, and 20% by the insured, of the next $1-2,000 in expenses. In other words, we paid the first $100, then 20% of the next $1,000 or so. The deductible plus the amount of co-insurance paid by the insured, is called the "out-of-pocket" expense.

Well, deductibles have increased (in order to lower premiums) to as high as $10,000 (I sold a policy with one) or more, and the average co-insurance limit is about $5,000. Co-insurance percentages have been adjusted and are now available at 70-30%, 60-40%, and even 50-50%, in another effort to lower premiums.

When insurance companies (casualty companies included) seriously entered into the health insurance market, there was a subtle change in the way expenses were covered. Whereas Blue Cross paid the hospital, and Blue Shield paid the doctor (in the hospital) and the deductible was only on the major medical (along with the co-insurance); insurance policies incorporated all the coverages into one, on which there was a deductible (and co-insurance) across the board. The calendar year was the time period on which the plan was based; with a consolation that the last three months of the previous year were included: this is called a carry-over provision and means that medical expenses incurred in October, November and December of a preceding year can be carried over to the current year; of course, if they weren't paid as claims in the preceding year.

Note: Insurance companies also sell "per cause" plans where the deductible is paid per sickness or accident and is good (usually) for six months, unless further treatment of the same or related illness is necessary, then the benefit period may be extended (six months at a time) for up to three years, or more. These are normally sold individually (non-group) and are harder to find than calendar year plans. They make more sense, in a catastrophic case, especially, because the benefit period starts when it is needed and lasts until it isn't, regardless of the time of year; but, they haven't won as much acceptance from the public, as calendar year plans.

So, the difference between Blue Cross/Blue Shield (including major medical) coverage and a health insurance policy from an insurance company is that Blue Cross is a pre-payment plan and is comprised of a membership of subscribers who (believe it or not) have voting privileges; while a health insurance policy is a legal instrument (contract) representing an

agreement with an insurer to cover a risk
(possible loss). Risk is more obvious in the
casualty business, and is usually accidental in
nature; for example: windstorm damage to a
house, or a car collision, etc.

The main problem with underwriting
health insurance is concerning "pre-existing
conditions"; another problem concerns "medically necessary treatment" on which there will
be more later.

Since the serious entry of the insurance
companies into health coverage, the Blues now
hold about 60% of the market share, and the
insurance companies about 40% – not including
health maintenance organizations (HMOs).
Because of this, the insurers have influenced
the Blues into becoming more like them in their
coverage. Most plans, now, have across-the-
board (hospital, doctors, etc.) deductibles on a
calendar year basis, with the three month
carryover allowance. Also, the Blues have
more participating (contracted) hospitals. In
the past, it was mandatory (if you were a Blue
Cross subscriber) to receive treatment at a
contracted ("Blue Cross") hospital which was
usually in your home area, to have full, or
sometimes, any coverage.

Insurance companies have treated health care as a risk, and did not stipulate where care had to be received (as long as the providers were licensed, etc.), only that it was based on reasonable and customary costs. These costs were eventually pinpointed to geographical areas, on which the premiums are based.

The Blues originally had schedules of costs for surgery and other medical procedures printed in their individual certificates, which were sent to subscribers. As costs by providers (hospitals, doctors, etc.) eventually increased, and at such a fast pace, they adopted *UCR*, which means usual, customary and reasonable; so that they wouldn't have to keep mailing out new certificates every time prices went up. Subscribers didn't seem to care, as long as the bill was paid, which until the Blues tried to control the providers, it usually was.

As health care costs (and premiums) continued to escalate, the Blues gave more attention to the providers, attempting to control the pricing of their services. As we have seen by the inflation in health care costs, they were not very successful. So, premiums increased and more people left the Blues, including large employers, and began to buy "health insurance" from insurers who were to glad to get the business.

One of the most motivating times for people to change was after they received a bill from the Blues explaining that they owed a balance (for services that had been received from providers), either because of a deductible and co-insurance, or because a provider didn't accept the UCR, set by the Blues: and the subscriber was responsible for the difference. Most people had stuck with the Blues through premium increases; but, having to pay in addition to what had been in their minds "full coverage" was the other barrel shot that began the revolution.

The problem with the business going to the insurers was that they were relatively new to the health care arena and had underestimated the potential costs involved. They were also somewhat spoiled, because most of them were life insurers, and life insurance had involved very little service (claims). So, as the claims started pouring in, the honeymoon was soon over. One good result of their being in the business was the development of (higher) deductibles; depending on your viewpoint, of course. The Blues had been reluctant to raise deductibles (or even have any) because their strength had been full coverage. The other advantage that the Blues had was "no claim forms" because of their relationships with the providers, especially hospitals.

By the way, the hospitals didn't make it easy for non-Blues customers. All the way down to the nurses and receptionists, the attitude was that if you didn't have "Blue Cross," things were going to be difficult for you. I think, part of this attitude was because of the newness of insurance plans, which meant more work (claim forms, interpreting coverages, etc.). Another part of the problem was the unfamiliarity with unheard of and out-of-state (alien) companies and their unknown ability or willingness to pay the patients' bills. The sick part was clinging to a decaying relationship and not having the good of people, in general, in mind. It was bad enough having to go to the hospital, and then having to deal with paranoia and resistance.

For all intents and purposes, the Blues are non-profit organizations, and are supposed to operate on a budget that breaks even at the end of their fiscal year. Most of them have a 5-10% administrative cost. The problem that occurs is that management tends to get complacent (in their relationship with providers) and as their salaries rise, in time with premium increases, they are less willing to "rock the boat." Obviously, they haven't been able to control spiralling health care costs.

The idea of having a third party which acts as a mediator between consumers and providers should have a levelling effect on the overall situation; even considering the administrative costs, as long as the third party does its job efficiently and productively. What were claim-handlers and premium collectors have now become watchdogs, because of increasing health care costs. They watch not only the providers (for abusive pricing); but, also potential policy owners (now, even subscribers to the Blues and HMOs) when they are seeking relief from high premiums by changing policies: pre-existing conditions are the major handicap in the free market process of purchasing health care coverage; especially, individual or small group plans (see Chapter 4, "Buying Health Insurance:" and Chapter 6 for more information on pre-existing conditions).

Historical Review (Footnotes)

1.   "In 1759 the Presbyterian Synod of Philadelphia established 'a Corporation for the Relief of Poor and Distressed Presbyterian Ministers and of Poor and Distressed Widows and Children of Presbyterian Ministers.'

2.   1929 – "A group of school teachers arranged for Baylor Hospital in Dallas, Texas to provide room and board and specified ancillary services at a predetermined monthly cost."
This was the forerunner of Blue Cross.

3.   1939 – "The first Blue Shield plan (Medical-Surgical), called the California Physicians' Service, was developed."

4.   1949 – "Major medical expense benefits were introduced by Liberty Mutual Insurance Company to supplement basic medical care expenses."

[1]"A Short History of Life Insurance" by Milfred F. Stone

[2]*Medical Care, Medical Costs* by Rashi Fein

[3,4]*Source Book of Health Insurance Data,* 1989:
Health Insurance Association of America.

CHAPTER 2 – USING YOUR HEALTH INSURANCE

Whether you are a Blue Cross subscriber or a policyholder (or certificate holder) with an insurance company, coverages are basically the same, assuming that you have "major medical" (most people do): all "medically necessary" treatment should be covered. If you have a hospital/surgical plan, you may want to take a close look at your policy, and pay closer attention to the "miscellaneous expense" coverage, if there is any. Today, with CAT-scans, MRIs and a lot of treatment being done on an outpatient basis, older hospital/surgical plans could be seriously lacking in coverage. If you belong to an HMO, you are pretty much in their hands.

The first concern to the consumer, in this case, subscriber or policyholder, is the deductible: almost all major medical plans, now have first-dollar deductibles, which means that the consumer pays the first dollars incurred as expenses. Some older plans, especially Blue Cross/Blue Shield, only had a deductible on the major medical expenses (doctor visits,

prescriptions and other expenses beyond the basic hospital/surgical coverage.
(see Chapter 1).

Some other older plans had a corridor deductible which occurred after the base plan had paid a certain amount in expenses, say $5,000. If you have an indemnity policy that only pays so much a day for a hospital room, and has a schedule for surgery; look for a cheap hospital and hope that you don't end up in intensive or coronary care.

OK, let's say that you do end up in the hospital; you don't pay the deductible right away. First the bill is compiled. Then the provider or the carrier (which could be the Blues, an insurance company, or even a health maintenance organization), *deducts* the first, say $250 which is what you owe. After the $250 is deducted, the next, say $4,000 is pro-rated according to the co-insurance feature of your coverage. If you have an 80/20% plan, then you would be responsible (possibly) for another $800, which is 20% of the $4,000.

Note: This is the way that you can tell that you have a "true" or "comprehensive" major medical plan, which is the best type of coverage (in spite of the deductible and the co-insurance). The reason it is better than the others is that it covers all your expenses (except, maybe the extra charge for a private room versus a semi-private room, and of course, television rental and telephone calls).

15

So, the total out-of-pocket cost that you have is $250 plus $800 or $1,050 which should be the maximum, regardless of how much the bill is or how much more that you have in medical expenses in that calendar year (up to the dollar limits of the plan – don't worry, most plans are $1-2 million lifetime with reinstatement provisions, annually – check it out, yourself.) Also, before you pay for your end of the expenses (assuming this is the first time that you have expenses *in excess* of your deductible during *this* calendar year) check back to the beginning of the year (January 1, almost always) for any other medical expenses that you may have paid, including: doctor visits (but usually not just physical examinations), prescriptions, crutches, or anything else that was medically necessary, treatment or supplies. You may also go back to October, November, and December of the previous year for the same things, unless they had been paid in that year. This is your carry-over period.

(Above) I just said that $1,050 is the maximum that you should pay – well, that is if everything that was "medically necessary" is reasonable and customary, or with the Blues, usual, customary and reasonable (UCR). The words are not important, or what order that they are in; in fact, they vary among carriers. What is important, however, is how much of a schedule they have.

The schedules, which can be called various things, including diagnosis-related groups (DRGs) for hospital costs, and prospective payment systems (PPSs) for doctors' costs for surgery and other services (both of these have been implemented by the federal government, in an effort to control Medicare reimburse-ments) are lists of costs that are to be expected for specified services in certain geographical areas. The carriers use these listings to verify claims that are presented. Most carriers want to keep their customers happy, or at least keep them from going to another carrier; so, most charges are deemed reasonable and customary, unless they are beyond borderline, or cause the claim-handler to be suspicious.

There are two exceptions to what would seem to be normal business behavior (above) – and the major one is the Blues. Because they have been doing schedules longer, and because they still have the lion's share of the market (60%, but the other 40% is divided among many insurance companies and then, the HMOs), they seem to have an attitude against paying what is above their UCR schedule.

The minor exception, although it can be expensive, is with anesthesiologists or anesthe-tists; for some reason, they keep charging more than what carriers deem to be reasonable and customary, especially Medicare. I don't know who is at fault here, but most of the complaints that I have had from my clients, in regard to bills that were not totally paid because of overcharges, have been in this area. Needless to say, the doctors feel that the schedules are too low; but, it's *your* problem.

If you get into a situation (pickle-in-the-middle) where the carrier has limited payment because of a UCR schedule, and the doctor is sending you nasty notices for the difference, don't panic: first, try to find out (if no one else has) if there is a reason for the extraordinary charge; for example: complications in surgery. The doctor's office should be co-operative and a local phone call away, and most carriers have toll-free numbers that you can call. If you are not inclined to this tactic, you can call your agent. As a last resort you can contact the insurance department in your state. Basically, there is no federal appeal – you might find a consumers group that would be interested: but, they, like lawyers, are not likely to be interested in these marginal cases.

As far as doctors' visits, prescriptions, etc., that you have paid during the year (or in the carry-over period); they can be used to satisfy your deductible and your co-insurance share, if you incur expenses, such as a hospital stay, and you are billed, as in the earlier example. In that case, before submitting payment of your end, send the bills that you have paid during the year, with a claim form, to your carrier.

Always make copies of what you send; and, if possible, try to get the name of the person who will be handling your file, and direct it to him or her, accordingly.

Sometimes carriers pay providers directly, sometimes they reimburse you – anything can happen. Usually hospitals are paid directly; when you sign the admittance form, you are assigning your insurance benefits to the hospital, for services provided. If you know that you will be going into the hospital – contact your carrier first (except for emergencies) to find out if you are subject to cost-containment or utilization review (more later).

If you don't go in the hospital, or don't have expenses that exceed your deductible on a particular occasion, save your bills, receipts, etc. for the year, and the last three months of the previous year. If, and/or when, the total exceeds your deductible, then submit them to your carrier.

Example: $300 in expenses submitted – deduct $250, then they reimburse you 80% for the next $50, or $40. By the way, always keep medical expenses on a per person basis when submitting claims. Use a claim form for each person, if you have more than one person, in the family, making claims; at least, until you have satisfied your family deductible.

The family deductible is usually two or three times the individual deductible, in other words, $500 or $750 per family, per year. It is possible to satisfy the family deducible without any member having $250 in expenses; and, if that happens, you will be reimbursed because of your co-insurance, at 80%, on expenses above the deductible.

Example: Three people in the family have $200 in expenses each, which equals $600 – deduct $500, then the carrier reimburses 80% of the next $100, or $80.

Some coverages have a "common" accident provision: if two or more members of the family are involved in a common accident, only one (or two) deductible(s) would apply, instead of two (or three); it is usually one deductible less than under ordinary circumstances. Some insurance policies, especially individual (non-group) ones, waive the deductible for any and all family members in the case of accidents (this is basically a built-in accident policy for the amount of the deductible).

Most major medical plans have "supple-mental" accident coverage which pays the first $300 or $500 (sometimes $1,000) of accident expenses on a per-accident basis. This coverage is in addition to the basic calendar year coverage on which the deductible is applied.

Usually there is a time limit for expenses: anywhere from 72 hours to 90 days on each accident; but I have never seen a limit on the number of accidents (per year or whatever). Also, it is first-dollar coverage and will pay up to the amount specified, so claims should be submitted as soon as possible: make sure that on the claim form that is submitted, that it is understood that it was an accidental injury; usually there is a box that can be checked off – put a big check, if not, attach a note. If the amount of the claim for an accident goes over the specific amount of the supplement, then the overage goes on your calendar year.

Example: If you have a $650 accident, and you have $500 in supplemental accident coverage; they pay the first $500, then $150 is covered by the major medical plan. So, if you have had no other expenses in that year to satisfy your deductible, then you pay the $150 which is then credited to your deductible. If you have had other expenses during the year, the overage ($150) would be added, just like any other expense for that calendar year; so, if your deductible was satisfied, you would only owe 20% of the $150, or $30. If your co-insurance limit had been reached, the $150 would be paid, or covered at 100%.

If you have a $300 accident, it would be paid in full, regardless of where you are in your major medical coverage (or calendar year).

21

Review of a hospital stay:
Total cost = $10,000:
You have a $250 deductible, then
80/20% of the next $4,000; you pay $250, then
20% of $4,000 or $800 plus $250 = $1,050 total.
You have satisfied your deductible and your
co-insurance limit and have reached your
maximum out-of-pocket; any additional expenses incurred during the rest of the calendar
year are paid by the plan at 100% (this assumes
that the providers' charges were reasonable
and customary). Any expenses paid before the
stay and in the same year, or the last 3 months
of the previous year (if not reimbursed) should
be submitted before final payment is made on
your part.

Example 2: Hospital stay
Total cost = $10,000:
(You have previous qualified expenses that you
have paid, of $200)
You have a $250 deductible, then 80/20% of the
next $4,000; you owe $250, then 20% of the next
$4,000 or $800 plus $250 = $1,050. You have
paid $200 during the year, so submit the paid
bills and $850, or just the paid bills, and you
will get a new bill for $850.

Example 3: Hospital stay:
Total cost = $2,250:
(You have previous qualified expenses that you have paid of $600)
You have a $250 deductible, then 80/20% of the next $4,000; you owe $250, then 20% of the next $2,000, or $400 plus $250 = $650. You have paid $600 during the year (assuming that these expenses were not claimed during the year), they should be submitted as soon as possible; claims are fed into the computer when they are received, although the service date is what the plan goes by – that is, the date on which you received treatment or the date that you entered the hospital. Also, it is very important that the claim-handler understands that the bills were paid by you. Usually this kind of a situation gets messed up; but, it doesn't have to, if the paperwork is clear and understandable. Remember that the person who is receiving your information, although he or she should be familiar with the process, does not understand your case, in particular, as well as you do. In other words, the chronological order isn't important, per se, but because you have paid in excess of your deductible, it can be confusing. The first bills (received) go to the deductible, then to the co-insurance, and so forth. The simplest thing to do here is to subtract the $600 that you have paid from the $650 that you owe; but, depending on how the bills are entered, and when, they may be paid at only 80%.

Example 4: Outpatient surgery:
Total cost $2,750.
(Assuming no other expenses during the year)
You have a $250 deductible, then
80/20% of the next $4,000; you pay the first
$250, then 20% of the next $2,500, or $500 plus
the $250 (deductible) equals $750 total. You
have satisfied your deductible (for the year)
and $2,500 of your co-insurance limit. The next
$1,500 in expenses will be covered on the 80/
20% basis. When and if, total expenses (for the
whole of the year) reach $4,250, then the plan
pays anything over $4,250 at 100% (instead of
80%).

Note: Some plans have a special feature
that pays 100% for outpatient surgery, to
encourage lower costs versus inpatient surgery;
others have incentives where you don't have to
pay the deductible, either. Usually it costs
more to have surgery in the hospital (either
inpatient or outpatient); because hospitals have
been charging more for outpatient surgery to
make up for the loss in revenue.

The least expensive option for outpatient
surgery is a free-standing surgical center.
These are beginning to appear instead of new
hospitals, as the need for bed-space declines
with the improvements in surgery. A lot of
surgery that would have required several days
in the hospital, in the past, can now be done on
an outpatient basis, especially laser surgery.

The best rule for submitting claims is:
Once you reach your deductible with doctor
visits, prescriptions, etc. submit those bills to
your carrier. If you submit them individually,
as they occur, it may give you some satisfaction
(you receive a statement saying that the
amount has been applied to your deductible);
but, it is a relatively expensive process. The
cost of handling a claim has been estimated at
about $15 per claim, so it's only economical
sense to save them up.

Another temptation, against common
sense, is duplication of coverage. This usually
occurs when both spouses work. Because of
the "co-ordination of benefits" clause in your
certificates (or policies) there is no advantage in
having double coverage: both companies
won't pay – even if they did, it wouldn't be
long before they found out, and you could
have a legal problem. Remember, we are living
in the information age, and computers can do
some amazing things.

Also, if you think the scenario in Example 3
was confusing, co-ordination of benefits is a
nightmare; neither carrier wants to have primary coverage, and they can go back and forth,
back and forth, and back and forth until you
are receiving not just nasty notes from doctors'
offices; but, threatening letters from collection
agencies, and experiencing fears of losing your
credit rating and other harassments. I had one

claim that took over a year to settle because of duplication of coverages. Pick out the best coverage for your situation and check with your employer, if it's your spouse's plan. If you have a cafeteria plan at work, there may be alternative benefits available to you; if not, I'm sure your honesty will be appreciated.

It's all right to have an individual indemnity plan to supplement your major medical coverage, to cover your deductible and co-insurance liability, but I'm not encouraging anyone to run out and buy one. What you would spend for a policy that would pay $50 a day for a hospital room, you would be better off saving, especially today. Hospital stays are getting shorter, on the average, less than a week; and the biggest expenses are not normally covered in this kind of a policy.

In review: The best thing to do is
1. Keep good records;
2. Make copies when you submit bills;
3. Deal directly with one person, if possible;
4. Submit claims on a per person basis;
5. Save the bills that have been paid during the year, and the last 3 months of the previous year; and
6. Be patient – the last time I heard, Blue Cross was 8 months behind in its payments to hospitals.

"PRE-CERTIFICATION/PRE-ADMISSION"
COST CONTAINMENT AND
UTILIZATION REVIEW

Last, but most important, today, is cost containment or utilization review. More and more coverage has these features. If you look at it from the health maintenance organizations' view, they have always had it. In other words, if you belong to an HMO, you have to go there, and they control their own expenses. From what I understand, most HMOs pay their doctors' salaries. I suppose that they would also receive some type of incentive or bonus, possibly profit-sharing or some arrangement like a retirement plan. Some HMOs have done well, especially *Kaiser Permanente*; many have started up, a lot have failed (more in Chapter 3).

Because most plans still offer the freedom of choice of providers (preferred provider organizations or PPOs are quasi-HMOs where a list of hospitals, clinics, doctors, etc. is used, see Chapter 3), some mechanism has become necessary to control health care costs on a broad scale, especially when schedules (UCR) haven't done the job.

Basically, cost containment (my favorite word for it) or utilization review (probably the original insurance company word for it) and there are many others like *Cost-Watch, Cost-Sentinel, Cost-Management*, etc. mean that before you spend any serious money, the carrier wants you to contact the reviewer first. In fact, most carriers specify time-periods in which you *must* contact them before certain procedures; an example would be: 10 days before a certain surgery. All the plans that I have seen exempt emergencies (then you have usually 48 hours afterwards to contact them, if possible). They also have toll-free numbers, usually on the I.D. cards.

The penalties (for not contacting them) range from 50% of the total benefits that you would have received (I'm not mentioning any names here, and there could be worse out there) under normal circumstances; which means if you would have contacted them and stayed the recommended days, etc., to a flat $100 (and there might be something less, like a slap on the wrist, but I haven't seen it yet).

If you are not familiar with cost containment or utilization review, and suspect that it applies to you, it is in your best interests to get more information: either from your employer, your agent, or a brochure from the insurer.

This has not been a very popular topic of conversation among intermediaries (brokers, agents, etc.) and even employers (if your plan is self-funded or self-administered).

Basically, the function of cost containment is the same as scheduling or UCR, except that it is done beforehand. Insurers are trying to get insureds more involved in the health care process. The best feature of utilization review is the avoidance of unnecessary surgery. It has been suggested (and as an agent listening to clients in the field, I believe it) that about half of the surgery performed in the United States is unnecessary. Both cost containment and utilization review are practically the same (as are the others) today, the names reflect the emphasis when they began (cost and use).

If you are contemplating surgery (unless it is very minor) you can expect to be requested to get a second opinion; and depending on the situation, you may be asked to get a third. Most plans have a list of surgeries that require pre-authorization in their brochures.*

They also may have an incentive benefit for second opinions; that is, they may pay 100% instead of 80%, which is not really a big deal, because it's very easy for major surgery to exceed most co-insurance limits, anyway.

---

*See *Appendix* (Odds and Ends) for a sample list of typical surgeries that require pre-authorization; but, contact the review organization, anyhow, even if it's minor surgery.

Some plans may even waive the deductible on second opinions, or provide a supplemental benefit equal to the cost.

The bottom line is that they are going to recommend not so much where you go (unless it is an HMO or PPO); but, if it's a hospital stay, for example, how long you stay; according to information that they have compiled which reflects averages for specific conditions or treatments.

They also can (and maybe will) tell you what the expected charges for surgery are, and their accompanying ancillary services.

If you malinger in the hospital, you may have to pay the additional expenses (for the extra days), and you could end up owing your doctor money, too.

CHAPTER 3 – CHOOSING YOUR HEALTH INSURANCE

Your choice depends mainly on your employer; unless you are paying for it yourself (see Chapter 4). If your employer has more than 25 employees, you should be able to choose between an HMO (health maintenance organization) and conventional insurance (Blue Cross included). If you work for an employer with 100 or more employees, you may have a cafeteria plan with several choices of health insurance plus other benefits, such as disability, dental, etc. Disability and dental plans are available to smaller groups; but, most companies have gotten away from them, or were never involved with them.

One of the ideas behind a cafeteria plan (which is what it sounds like -- you choose from a spread of what is available) is to offer employees, who have spousal coverage for their health insurance, something to use as compensation for not enrolling in *their* plan. Basically, the smaller that the employer is, the less choice that you will have; although you may have more input (with a smaller employer) as to what plan the company installs.

If you choose an HMO, you will have to use their doctors, facilities, etc.; but, you will probably have a lower (maybe zero) deductible than with the insurance-type (conventional) plan. HMOs usually have arrangements with local hospitals (if necessary) and other doctors (usually specialists); but the option of using them is up to the HMO. What it means to them, of course, is an additional cost (even though it may be discounted) if they need to send you elsewhere. They also have provisions for emergencies: if you like to travel, you should check these out very carefully (especially if you travel out of the United States).

With an insurance-type plan you should be able to use any hospital (licensed) of your choice, unless it's a PPO (preferred provider organization) which will furnish you with a list of providers that are involved (members).

Some plans are a mixture of conventional insurance and a PPO -- if you go to a non-member hospital or doctor you will pay a standard deductible and co-insurance amount; but, if you go to a member provider, you will have a reduced deductible and/or co-insurance amount. These plans are relatively new and can be confusing if you mix member and non-member providers. The idea behind a PPO is to allow some choice and still control costs by an internal agreement among the providers.

As far as claims are concerned -- an HMO handles all its own paperwork which is reduced by not having a third party such as Blue Cross or an insurer (insurance company, third-party administrator or self-insured employer's mediator). In other words, you are pretty much like a member of a club, and if your dues are paid, you are entitled to the benefits it has to offer. One of the advantages of a PPO, because of its organization, should be in handling claims. If done properly, it should shift the burden of the paperwork, which should be standardized, from the claimant (consumer) to its own organization. The conventional insurance plans still require claim forms, although most hospitals, and more doctors, are internalizing the process through their own offices by assignment (the claimant assigns his/her benefits over to the provider who receives payment directly from the insurer).

Prescriptions

If prescriptions are of concern to you (and at today's prices they should be) an HMO with a pharmacy will probably have the lowest deductible or least out-of-pocket expense, possibly none. Most have plans where you would pay, say $2, for a regular prescription, or $1 for its generic equivalent. PPOs should have member pharmacies and cost a little more, but this can vary widely (information regarding deductibles and details should be available to you).

Conventional insurance plans (including Blue Cross) have covered prescriptions since the advent of major medical coverage in the 1950's; but, most of those covered didn't (or don't) know it, and the companies didn't (or don't) go out of their way to inform them. (I didn't even know Blue Cross, with major medical, covered prescriptions until I overheard a conversation in a restaurant between two subscribers, back in the early 1980's.) Of course, prescription expenses are subject to your calendar year deductible (and co-insurance) which was $100 (and 80/20% of the next $2,000) then.

Most group plans offer a prescription card, for a premium in addition to the health insurance coverage. There are some good stand-alone (sold separately) plans; but, they are very expensive, unless there is a large group involved (100 or more employees). A typical mini-group (under 20 employees) plan through a national carrier, with a $5 (average) deductible will cost a family of four (male age 40, female age 40 and two children) about $48 a month (more on buying health insurance in Chapter 4).

Mail-order plans are gaining popularity with group insurers who have experienced high costs with drug cards, or even as major medical claims; as prices escalate on prescriptions. Orders are placed with a code number that is furnished by the insurer. This establishes you as a member, and either entitles you to a discounted price, or access with a per order fee and/or prescription deductible (so far, about the same as a drug card). These plans vary significantly but usually have one national provider. The obvious problem is with drugs that you need right away. Also, some drugs cannot be sent in winter (cold weather) when there is a danger of them freezing. I imagine some can't be sent when it's too hot, but (being in northern Ohio) I wouldn't know about that; although, it is getting warmer here.

In Conclusion & *C.O.B.R.A.*

These are basically the plans that are available; but, unless you have a cafeteria plan (25 or more employees for automatic HMO option), you won't be able to pick or choose. In fact, most plans require all employees to participate. If not, the insurers face the problem of adverse selection, or "carve-out" which is when only the people with bad teeth take the dental plan, or only those seeking early retirement take the disability plan.

If you have a choice, for example, between an HMO or a PPO or a conventional plan, a lot is going to depend on the location(s) of the provider(s) in the HMO or PPO. If drugs are free at the HMO; but, it costs more in gas to get there, than the deductible on a mail-order plan (which, by the way, usually sends 60-90 day supplies) and you can't wait a few days for a new supply, etc...well, you can see the dilemma with prescription coverage.

The main concern that you should have is; if you became seriously ill where would you (and family members) be comfortable being treated, especially if you had to make frequent visits before or after a hospital stay?

If you *lose* your health insurance because you leave an employer (and don't have a spouse with coverage) you will probably be interested in the next chapter; but, before you run out and buy something, you may have an option (for a while) to the market place. If your employer (ex-employer, by now) has 20 or more employees left (usually this means full-time and year-round); you should be able to continue your old coverage (without changes) at the same price, which *you* would have to pay, plus (possibly) a 2% per month handling charge. You may do this for 18 months, and under certain circumstances up to 3 years (dependents are included); because of C.O.B.R.A., the Consolidated Omnibus Budget Reconciliation Act of 1986; C.O.B.R.A. guidelines:

The 18 month continuation option; when coverage would end due to:

- Reduction in work hours
- Voluntary termination
- Lay-off for economic reasons
- Discharge for misconduct
(except gross misconduct).

The 36 month continuation option:

· Children of current employees who lose eligibility because of age (usually 19, unless full-time students)
· Surviving spouses/children of deceased employees
· Separated, divorced, or Medicare ineligible spouses and children of current employees.

If you want to continue your coverage, you have *60 days* to let your employer know.

O.B.R.A., the <u>O</u>mnibus <u>B</u>udget <u>R</u>econciliation <u>Act</u> which was passed later in 1986 includes C.O.B.R.A. coverage for retirees and their spouses and dependents of companies undergoing Chapter 11 Reorgnization.

Chapter 4 – Buying Health Insurance; the Deductible

Without tooting my horn too much -- I have made a living selling health insurance (exclusively) for the last ten years: this advice comes from my experience in Ohio and western Pennsylvania; but should apply to any part of the country.

First of all, for those who don't already know: the higher the deductible is, the lower the premium will be: everything else being equal. The way to look at the deductible is as something that you will have to pay if you incur medical expenses up to that amount.

When I started selling health insurance, I sold a hospital policy (with surgical and miscellaneous benefits) which was designed to replace Blue Cross/Blue Shield. The people that I called on then were paying about $200 a month (a family) for the Blues, and basically had full coverage, in the hospital. We had a policy that offered basically the same coverage, except for maternity; but, had a $500 deductible with no co-insurance. In other words, if you went into the hospital, you owed the first $500, then everything else was paid 100% by the company. This type of plan originated in Florida as "quick-pay" but was marketed out of Dallas, through a national small business association.

The presentation logic was really simple: because the premium was $50 a month cheaper ($150 for a family), the main question was, "Mr. and Mrs. Jones, how often do you go into the hospital?". Most men hadn't gone at all, and most women had gone only for maternities (most of the people that I visited with were not interested in having more children -- they were usually older, small-business owners). The next statement was, "If you save $50 a month for 10 months, then you will have $500, which is your deductible! Do this for each family member, over time, and you are ahead of the game."

Things have become more complicated since then; but you can apply the same mathematics in other cases; for example: if the difference in premium between a $500 deductible and a $1,000 deductible is $50 a month -- your liability is increased $500; but, you save $50 a month. The biggest problem with health insurance (other than with pre-existing conditions) is that you don't know what will happen in the future (no crystal ball). Some say insurance is a gamble -- insurance companies don't like to be thought of as casinos, however, and argue accordingly.

However you want to look at it, if you are going to expose yourself to a risk (a loss), the deductible is the best place to do it. It is better to have a high deductible on a plan that covers catastrophic expenses, than it is to have no deductible on a policy that has unrealistically limited benefits (five years ago, the average cost for heart surgery at the Cleveland Clinic was over $50,000). Without becoming para-noid, I think it's best to assume the worst, and pay the little bills ($200-300 a year) for doctor's visits, etc., yourself, out of the money that you save with a higher deductible.

This economic philosophy isn't popular, as most people like to see the insurer reimburse them occasionally, but that's really a psycho-logical problem. Also, the more paperwork that is involved, the more expensive the premiums will be, in general. Another thing is: people with lower deductibles use their benefits more often, therefore their rates are proportionately higher. Today, with the use of computers, rates are pretty much based on statistical usage, allowing for a little creative marketing. Insurers like high deductibles and should reflect this in their premium schedules (rates).

It's hard for us to like deductibles, when *we* have to pay them. But think of what the chances are of incurring a really large medical expense. Most expenses are affordable, even though they are aggravating to pay -- what you really need is protection for the "catastrophic loss"- you may not be able to get the treatment that you want or need without it, or you may have to go "broke" in the process. (Medicaid later).

If you can't get excited about a high deductible, and anticipate a lot of smaller expenses, and possibly maternities -- your best bet, financially, would be a health maintenance organization (HMO), if you find one in your area that would be convenient to you and your family. As explained in earlier chapters, HMOs should be cheaper than conventional insurance-type plans; but, they will not have the choice of providers. Preferred provider organizations (PPOs) don't discount premiums that much, but should mean less out-of-pocket expense (deductible and co-insurance). Blue Cross has always had the best maternity coverage: most insurers offer decreased benefits for normal maternities versus "any other illness or injury coverage"; but, complications of pregnancy are automatically included in all health insurance coverage, by Federal mandate.

The situation should dictate the coverage. If you are a healthy older couple without dependent children, for example: you don't need a traditional family plan with maternity (unless you want to start another family -- many people still have these). The exception would be an old policy, providing good coverage, that was less expensive than a new plan. Your coverage should be tailored to your needs/wants and your budget, currently. If you have a large or growing young family, and the local HMO is agreeable to you, geographically and otherwise, move in!

Most insurance plans that are offered today are step-rated. This means that the premium is based on the insured's sex and age, except for minor children that are dependent (then it will be based on how many of them -- usually there is a limited premium of three, possibly four, regardless of how many more). On most individual (non-group) and some small group plans, you can get a discount if you are a non-smoker (you must not have smoked cigarettes, sometimes "not used any tobacco" for at least 12 months) which amounts to usually 10%, growing to 15% on some newer plans.

The older you are, the more that the premium is. Female rates are higher than males in the younger (19-50) years, without maternity; and the male rates are higher, later (50-65); they are almost even around age 50. Medicare applies to those over age 65, unless you are disabled, before then; and the premiums drop significantly because of its coverage....(Chapter 8).

Again, the rates are based on experience, and the insurers have the statistics and the computers to use them, accordingly. Also, rates, nowadays, are based on attained or current age. In the past, as was the custom with life insurance, the nearest birthday was used for age; so, you will be better off applying for a policy a few weeks before your birthday, than a few days after. This is becoming more true with life insurance, too; but, there is no "back-dating to save age" with health insurance -- in fact, even if the application is dated before a birthday; but, the underwriting decision isn't made until after the birthday, the later date may be used, it's up to the company.

This is especially true when medical information is being requested from attending physicians, and received sometime in the process. In other words, an agent can submit an application and ask for the date when it was signed; but, he/she cannot bind coverage or guarantee anything. The agent can request a date (specific day of the month, up to the 28th) to coincide with your premium payment (monthly is almost always check-o-matic or bank-o-matic on individual policies -- that is the insurer takes the money out of your checking account automatically every month, on that day). If you don't like check-o-matic, you will probably have to pay at least quarterly, or semi-annually, or annually, if you are lucky; in which cases, the company will then bill you for subsequent premiums.

Note: If a company doesn't offer an annual premium, it is probably because they are planning to raise your rates before then -- in fact, probably more than what they could make on it, interest-wise. There are two reasons for check-o-matic: one is the expense of sending out bills every month for premiums versus the automatic transfer of funds; the other is that the business is more "persistent" when premiums are drawn automatically, especially monthly.

With few exceptions, the initial premium is submitted with the application for insurance, although it is refundable if you don't keep the policy: you should have at least 10 days , and up to 30 days (mandatory for Medicare supplements) to look over the policy and decide if you want to keep it. On individual policies, you should also have a 31 day grace period for paying premiums. It's interesting that I have never seen a grace period stated on a group plan (or certificate); but, companies will usually give the group up to 45 days to keep the plan in force, sometimes 60 days. The problem with not having a specified grace period is that, if you are late, the carrier (insurer) can deny any claims that are made in the late period by cancelling your coverage, that is not accepting the late ("untimely") premium.

Individual policies also have more protection rate-wise: they are usually controlled by state laws. All the policies of the same type that are issued by an insurance company in that state are treated as a "class" or block of business. In order to get a rate increase, the company has to present an accounting of the premiums collected against the claims that were paid to those policyholders. If the claims exceed the premiums by 20%, chances are that is what the increase will be. This is also true for association plans; but, they have some loopholes which make it easier for them to raise rates, and also to enter markets.

Group plans of less than 20 employees are normally not true groups. Depending on the carrier's definition, "true group" may require 50 or more employees on board. My definition of a true group is one that requires no medical information on enrolling employees (either current or future). In other words, it is a complete take-over of benefits ("no gain or no loss") of a group, "as-is or as-will-be," including any portions of calendar year deductibles that have been satisfied. New employees would be covered upon employment without a waiting period. This is an ideal definition, or a target which an employer may not be interested in hitting, because of the costs associated with the risks; so, many aberrations are offered in the marketplace.

Small group plans (less than 50 or so employees) that are not "true groups" may be anything from individually underwritten and ridered like individual policies to near the above "ideal".

CHAPTER 5 – EXCLUSIONARY RIDERS, AND AGENTS

Riders, or exclusions, are what insurers put on policies (individual) or certificates (group) to deal with pre-existing conditions; that is, if they want to cover the rest of your body (and mind), or in a group situation where they don't want to decline an applicant, entirely. A simple example is a hernia -- if you had been treated for a hernia within the last, say two years; the insurer might exclude coverage for "hernia (usually, the same particular area of the body) and complications thereof or therefrom," for probably six months. This is what the underwriters actually do, in health insurance. A complex example would be if you are taking medicine for high blood pressure (hypertension): to be covered at all, you might not mind the insurer excluding coverage for your prescriptions or doctors' visits; but, what about the complications thereof or therefrom?

Actually a rider can be anything at all that is added to a policy, including a benefit, such as supplemental accident coverage; but be aware of the language that is used and the specific time period, if there is one. By the way, all time, in health insurance, is based on the *effective date* of the policy, not the application date or the date of the check you signed to pay the initial premium.

Other language that you should look for in the policy (especially individual) is "major medical," or "comprehensive major medical" or even "major medical expense" (see Chapter 1). The words "major medical" define the policy as covering any "medically necessary" treatment above and beyond basic hospital and surgical-medical coverage.

There aren't any legal precedents in regard to this language, that I know of, and it is more a matter of custom and common usage; so, unless you want to set a precedent through the court system, read *all* the language in the policy. Policies are supposed to be easier to read and understand today, and I'd say that they are easier.

Most mini-groups (less than 20 employees for my purposes here -- 20 or more employees meet C.O.B.R.A. guidelines; see Chapter 3) are placed in "trusts". These have been traditionally called "multiple employer trusts" or METs, and originally were marketed to groups that had trouble getting coverage; because of hazardous occupations, seasonal employment cycles, etc., or not enough enrolling employees, for a true group. They were not as specific as trade associations, and generally were offered to broader groups, such as retailers. The trust operators were the modern pioneers of third-party administration. They developed a policy with an insurance company, and marketed it accordingly; they might handle the claims, as well.

The problem (although it has not been one, in general) is that you are "trusting" them to do well. The Trust is the policyholder, the group's participants receive certificates. This is a nominal difference, but it demonstrates the relationship. This can be a more economical and even more expeditious situation, depending on the efficiency and productivity of the trust; but, if the trust has problems, the groups might end up dealing with the insurer, and not under the most favorable circumstances. The best "policy" is dealing directly with the insurer (actually its agents) in the beginning. This does not mean dealing with "captive agents," necessarily.

Whom to Buy From

Captive agents are those who are contracted with one company. It is possible that one of them may have the best deal for you; but, they often sell other products for that company (mainly auto, home, or even, life insurance) and many are not very knowledgeable about health insurance, which is a different animal. Some people have a tendency to put all their "insurance eggs" into one basket; probably because they either like or trust their agent, or both. This is understandable, and it may even make economical sense, because of discount incentives for more than one policy (having multiple policies) with one carrier. For example: We can get a 10% discount on the car insurance because we have the house insured with the same company. It seems like everybody (and their sister) has been selling health insurance, lately; but, casualty companies (home, auto, etc.) are the newest source of entrants to the marketplace, and their agents are the least experienced with it.

A broker is an agent who deals with companies that do not ordinarily have captive agents. Usually referred to as "independent agents," they might not be that independent (just like Blue Cross administrators, relationships can develop); but, they should be able to offer you some good choices. Try to find a broker who "specializes" in health insurance (life insurance is usually on the same license, so be forewarned). A good broker can tailor a plan (they still vary) and a premium (price) to meet your wants/needs. If the broker keeps pushing one particular company, this is a symptom of a relationship that is in his/her best interests; although, not necessarily bad for you. Commission rates still vary, but they are becoming more homogenous; although bonuses for production are playing a larger role in steering business to certain companies.

Commissions on individual policies are higher in the first year, as an incentive to create new business (but dwarf in comparison to life insurance – which is why your agent is always trying to replace your policy). Renewals (second year and thereafter, commissions) decrease to what is called a service fee, eventually, which amounts to a few percent of the premium. Most small group plans are commissioned at about 10% of the premium. Larger group plans scale commission percentages down, in very large cases the commission could be less than 1%; because the more cumulative (based annually) premium, the lower the commission percentage. In other words, a group might start out paying 7%; but, as the total premium exceeds a certain amount (say $10,000) the commission percentage decreases (maybe 6%); another $10,000, and then it's 5%, and so on -- until renewal time, then it starts all over again at the higher rates.

Chapter 6 – Why Individual, and Why Not?

(Including Pre-Existing Conditions)

If you have a very small group (2-5 employees) and they are basically healthy, your best course of action would be to find individual coverage directly with an insurer (not a third-party administrator, or TPA). The entry (or street) rates should be about the same as a small group plan, and you are not required to buy life insurance. They usually offer options, such as maternity and supplemental accident, which are built into most group plans. Be aware that some states have laws requiring maternity coverage when you have a certain number of employees (in Ohio, you only need to have five employees to be liable for maternity expenses, even if you *don't* offer health insurance).

These laws stem from the original *Discrimination Acts of 1967*, however weirdly, which reminds us to make sure that everybody ("eligible employee") has the same coverage. You can vary the amounts of life insurance, if you choose to include it, according to classes of employees which you can define; but, don't discriminate within them. The same theory should apply to deductibles, but a reimbursement plan (in line with class of employee) would be easier to administer, and account for, in regards to employee compensation and Section 89 (more later).

Individual plans typically have premium increases with age, usually on the anniversary of the effective date of the policy; but, in recent history, these increases have been less than the "trend" (inflation index of health care costs) increases have been, and they have occurred less often than with groups. A lot of group plans are increasing premiums every 6 months. The current "trend" is about 2% a month, or around 24% a year. According to the rule of 72 for compound interest, at 24% a year, rates would double in 3 years (72 ÷ 24 = 3). Hopefully, health care inflation will decrease again – it was down to about 15% a year, a few years ago; and is showing signs, from the latest figures (see Appendix), of relief.

If you have a small group (and are able to get coverage) individual policies offer more flexibility in the future. If one of the employees develops a health problem and has a pre-existing condition from it, and the premiums are getting expensive (relative to new coverage) your group is not locked in with that carrier. You can leave the employee with his/her coverage, and the rest of you can get new policies. Also, if the unhealthy employee leaves your group, he/she can continue his/her coverage (without changes) on his/her own.

In other words, there are no participation requirements which you almost always have in group plans. Most group plans will allow for spousal coverage, and will let (maybe) 1 out of 4 employees waive coverage (for other good reasons); guidelines will vary with carriers.

Note to the employer: Always have any employee who is not being covered sign a waiver form and keep a copy for your records – it is for your protection.

Note to employees: always let your employer know if there is a change, in regard to a waiver; if your spouse no longer covers you because of work, etc.

If you have a small group (5-10 employees) it will be harder to get clean (without exclusionary riders) individual coverage, unless you are all very healthy. Also, you are more likely to want maternity benefits which are usually better in group plans. Basically, the more employees (therefore premium) that you have, the more likely the underwriters will be willing to bend (until you have around 5 employees, the underwriting is about the same as individual – except for "guaranteed issue"). It used to seem more glamorous to have "group coverage," and it *was* better in the past; but, there are very good individual policies available, today.

"Guaranteed issue" means that the insurance carrier will automatically cover eligible employees (from as few as two) enrolling in the plan (with strict participation requirements) but; will exclude "pre-existing conditions." The definition of "pre-existing" will vary, by time periods, with the carrier. Typically, a pre-existing condition is anything that was treated within the last two years (for smaller groups) or in the last 12 months (for larger groups). Treatment includes taking medication, visiting the doctor and getting advice or whatever. Sometimes language in this clause will state that, even if you didn't receive treatment or advice, that you should have been a "prudent

person," and if you knew or felt that something was wrong with you, that you should
have sought treatment.

Once *that* time period is established (from
the effective date of coverage, backwards) you
have your "pre-existing condition." The next
time period relates to when that condition will
be covered. Usually, it will be covered after 12
months (again, "on the plan," or from the
effective date of coverage.). Some plans will
cover a pre-existing condition after 6 months
(on the plan), if no further treatment (including
medicine or advice) is received, "on the plan."

In other words, if you were treated for
something 8 months before the effective date of
coverage and continue treatment through the
effective date, you will be covered 6 months
after the treatment stops, or at least in 12
months, from the effective date. If you received treatment before the effective date (in
the defined time period) but, not after the
effective date, the condition would be covered
in 6 months (and possibly a day, if you want to
be technical); check the language out in the
offer (rider).

Individual policies spell out the time periods and usually have specific language in the
riders (which are part of the policy). Underwritten (no guaranteed issue) small-group
plans should also make a specific reference to a

pre-existing condition and its time limit. The longest period of time for an exclusion should be 2 years. If there is no reference to time (in the rider, or in the overall language regarding pre-existing conditions) then it is probably what is called a "permanent" rider. These riders can usually be removed after 2 years, if no further treatment has been received (exceptions would be heart, liver, kidney, aneurism or lung problems, or internal cancers, etc.).

The reason I say two years is, that on an individual policy (or underwritten group plan), the insurance company can contest against fraud on an application. This is called a "contestability period" and lasts for 2 years from the effective date of coverage.

In other words, if you lie to them, by omitting something on the application, they can rescind your coverage in the first two years. Also, once you have not received treatment for two years (except serious conditions), you are probably ok, and your carrier knows that another carrier would probably pick you up without a rider. Now, I'm not encouraging anyone to omit things on the application and hold their breath for two years (because of this knowledge.).

Underwriters appreciate information, especially about your pre-existing conditions; and the more that you give them, the more likely you are to get a favorable offer, and a quicker response. By the way, a response to an application with pre-existing conditions can be delayed when information is requested from your doctor (attending physician's statement or APS) which, if information is lacking on the application, is more likely to be done.

This contestability period is a relative of one that is found in life insurance policies which excludes suicide. In fact, one of the exclusions of health coverage, usually after "acts of war" is self-inflicted injuries. Other exclusions are: cosmetic or elective surgery, treatment by a non-qualified provider or relative, dental work (except when caused by an accident), treatment covered by a government (Veterans' Administration, etc.) or Workers' Compensation, routine physicals, experimental treatments, corrective lenses, hearing aids, etc. Read a (your) policy sometime, it's interesting.

(See Appendix – General Exclusions, for longer list).

Some small (less than true) group plans offer an allowance for pre-existing conditions (not covered under the plan). Some are underwritten and specific about the provision. Guaranteed issue plans are more general: once a group is in force (coverage has started) pre-existing conditions are covered; but, for limited amounts. For example: a group of five employees may receive an allowance of $5,000 per calendar year (for all pre-existing conditions) or $2,000 per employee (per year) or possibly $1,000 per condition.

The language varies and can be confusing, often ambiguous. If you are interested in this type of plan, because of pre-existing conditions in your group, carefully consider the consequences, and the cost of possible treatment (it's usually more than you can imagine). When understood properly, and depending on the conditions, this can be a good alternative, though.

If you are not comfortable with the allowance, or just unhappy with insurance companies, it would be worth your while to check with your local Blue Cross; although they have been requiring more information, and more often decline applicants altogether (no riders). Some Blue Cross organizations are requiring physicals, especially for individual subscribers, and most have 3 and 6 month waiting periods, after you are accepted; first for Blue Cross (hospital coverage) and then Blue Shield (medical-surgical). With the Blues, make sure you are also getting "major medical" (Chapter 1) or, at least, "catastrophic coverage," and read the outline of coverage, and any schedules or provisions, such as waiting periods between confinements, etc. The brochures are usually very "sweet and simple" and tempting; but the Blues can be very complicated.

Some Blues' plans accept subscribers only at certain times (maybe in January, and then in July, or just one month) of the year. By the way, insurance carriers are beginning to require paramedical examinations (done at your home or office, at your convenience) which may include blood and/or urine samples (they don't usually say so; but, it's because of AIDS and drug abuse, mostly).

If (or when) you become frustrated with the Blues (it may be an ordeal just getting a hold of someone who can sell you something; Blue Cross is being sold by brokers, in some areas; but, usually not individual, only group); then it's time for the health maintenance organization, or HMO. By the way, Blue Cross group plans (2 or more, or you might need 10 or more employees) are almost the same, now, as insurance plans, and they may be even pickier in their underwriting.

HMOs are starting to get picky, also; but, they may be your best bet, if you are generally in good health even though you have had health problems in the past. With the HMOs, it is more a situation of timing, and of supply and demand: when you apply is important. They will probably require an application (with health history) and maybe a physical, depending on them, at the time. If you are not in real bad shape (relative to their current role versus their ability to provide service) you might get in during their normal year (of 11 months). If you can't get in one HMO and others are available, try them. If that doesn't work, there is one consolation, and at this point, it is very important.

HMOs are required (by charter) to have at least one *open* enrollment period per year (usually one particular month). The timing varies with the HMO, and you should be able to find it out from them; maybe, with a little pressure. If you can't find out, there should be a list of HMOs available which includes their open enrollment periods. This list should be available from your state insurance department, consumers' services division.

If you can't afford an HMO, or even an insurance policy with a high deductible, you might want to find out if you are eligible for Medi*caid*, from your Social Security office (Medi*care* is for those over 65, or who are disabled before then). See Chapter 8 – From Medicare to Medicaid.

Chapter 7 – Is It Cancellable? Or Re-Enterable?

Most states require that health insurance sold in their state is non-cancellable. Unfortunately, it is impossible for them to control every policy that is sold, and the problem usually isn't discovered until it's too late (after a claim or a cancellation). What you want to look for are the words "guaranteed renewable" or "*not* or *non*-cancellable by the insurer, for any reason except the payment of a premium." Auto insurance is cancellable and for good reasons, especially in states where a minimum amount of liability (for damage to others' property) is required to keep a driver's license and/or get license plates; but, it would be cruel and unusual punishment to cancel someone's health insurance, because he or she got sick or had an accident that caused bodily injury to themselves through no direct fault of their own.

In states that allow cancellable health insurance to be sold, you might have to search a little, and non-cancellable coverage (all else being equal) will be more expensive. When weighing the difference in premium, it is important to keep this in mind: if you have a large claim, and the company cancels you (hopefully after they pay it) you will probably have a "pre-existing" condition, and not be able to get new coverage from another carrier (let alone, another insurance company). Even if you attempt to hide the condition (by not disclosing it on the application) chances are that the new company will pick it up from the Medical Information Bureau, which is a service that collects and reports medical information, from and to insurance companies. The insurers have to pay for this service (around $30 per Social Security number) but; they are using it more and more. Also, new coverage will have a new contestability period (2 years again) for fraud.

Cancellability has been more of a problem with individual coverage, and because of this, many states have laws protecting individual policyowners. Also, small groups that are in (most) trusts may not be cancelled individually; but, there is little (or no) protection against rate (premium) increases, in trusts.

True groups (20-50 or more employees,
depending on the insurer) have no problem, as
long as they meet the required number of
employees; because "true group" (by definition) does not demand medical information on
the applicants (enrolling employees), so pre-
existing conditions are not a factor. It can be a
problem if you leave a group, though. If the
group has 20 or more employees, you should
be able to continue your coverage for 18
months, possibly 3 years under C.O.B.R.A.
(Chapter 3) (unless you leave because of gross
misconduct; also, you will have to pay the
premiums yourself). If you leave a group of
less than 20 employees, you may be offered a
conversion policy which usually offers less
coverage for more premium, which can be a
real dilemma, especially if you are not well
enough to work, or disabled. If you are disabled, and it is work-related, check with Workers' Compensation in your state; if they can't
help you, or it is not work-related, check with
Social Security.

"Guaranteed renewable" does not mean
forever; first, a company could go out of business – this is unusual and unlikely because of
financial reserves that are required of insurers;
but, as witnessed by the savings and loan
scandals, there are still a lot of manipulators
out there. Second, "guaranteed renewable"
means that an insurance company cannot

single out a policyholder because of claims presented (and assumingly paid), either by quantity or quality; but, what a company *can* do is to "not renew" for *all* of the same policies (in force) in the entire state.

Non-renewing has happened only in the last few years, and very minimally, although "non-renewing" has sponsored new coverage that is guaranteed to be guaranteed renewable. The language is a little confusing – what it means is that we pay a little more premium and get a little more peace of mind: more money goes into reserves to soften possible harder times in the future. So, if they go broke, they can't "not renew," they just go out of business, which, in most cases, results in a takeover by another insurer.

If companies start falling like dominoes (this is much less likely than the savings and loan thing) then we've all got problems, and probably higher taxes: Congress will think of something like some *more* laws, to bail us out.

If you belong to an HMO and it goes out of business (a lot do) and you can't find another to join in you area, you have got a double problem (with a pre-existing condition). First, as we know by now, insurance policies are underwritten, and a policy will be difficult to get if you have a health problem; even becoming a subscriber to Blue Cross/Blue Shield can be difficult. The other problem is that insurance companies don't like HMOs, and if you are trying to get new (individual) coverage, one of the questions on most applications is "Do you currently have (or have had) coverage?". Having belonged to an HMO (especially an extinct one), in this case, is probably worse than having had no coverage. With group plans (less than true) it becomes a problem when they ask "Who is (or was) your (previous) carrier?". It can even be a problem to a (near or just) true group, if a lot of employees had been enrolled in the HMO, that went out of business; because the HMO people could be treated as late applicants (to the existing insurance plan, if there is one).

"Late entry" or "late applicant" can, and usually does, result in medical underwriting. Even in the case of a true group (a very large group without the employees who have been in the HMO) it is possible for the insurer to require medical information on the applicants. In other words, insurance companies don't like it when an employee doesn't join their plan when it becomes effective, or if later, when the employee becomes employed (taking into consideration any waiting period set by the employer).

Example: ABC Company has 100 eligible employees: Because the number of employees is over 20, ABC has to offer HMO coverage, in addition to a conventional insurance plan. ABC's insurance company offers ABC a true group (no underwriting) plan; but, requires 70% participation or 70 employees (by their standards) to put it in place. 75 employees sign up for the insurance plan, 25 employees join the HMO. In this case, this is all done at the same time, say February 1. The HMO goes out of business later in the year, say October 1, and there is no other HMO to take over the business. The employees that joined the HMO want to sign up for the conventional plan; but, technically they are late entrants (because they didn't sign on February 1) and can be subjected to medical underwriting (an application, a physical, etc.).

The same problem exists when an employee doesn't sign up for a plan upon employment. A reason (and not a good one, as far as the insurance company is concerned) might be that he/she does not want to pay his/her part of the premium on a contributory plan (100% participation is usually required on non-contributory plans, that is when the employer pays the whole premium). If the employee tries to sign up "late," questions are undoubtedly going to be asked. Again, insurance companies are very wary of adverse selection – in this case (maybe) waiting until you are ready to go into the hospital, before buying health insurance; you're guilty until you prove yourself innocent.

CHAPTER 8 – FROM MEDICARE TO MEDICAID
(SUPPLEMENTS AND LONG TERM CARE)

Medicare and Medicaid were established by Social Security in 1965 as "supplemental" insurance for the disabled and aged (Medicare), and grants of medical assistance to the impoverished (Medicaid). On July 1, 1966, Medicare was expanded and became the main coverage for those aged 65 or older, unless they kept working for an employer who covered them. (Medicare is optional to groups of 20 or more employees – when you become eligible and are still working, or your spouse is working – you can accept or reject the employer plan).

"If you accept the employer plan it will be the primary payer of your hospital and medical bills and Medicare will be the secondary payer. This may pay a portion of any unpaid charges for services covered by

Medicare. If you do not accept your (or your spouse's) employer plan, Medicare will be the primary payer of any covered health services and supplies you receive. When Medicare is the primary payer, the employer plan is not permitted to pay supplemental benefits for Medicare-covered services."
Guide to Health Insurance for People with Medicare, 1990.

It is very expensive to keep seniors on a company plan as normal employees (full-time/ eligible). Insurers do not want to have what is called "primary" coverage on anyone aged 65 or older, because of the higher risks and costs that are associated with them, even when they are working full-time; therefore, the premiums are very high.

Lately, the federal government has been trying to force those who are working (and/or eligible for an employer plan because of a working spouse) to maintain that coverage. This saves Medicare (money) because the employer's insurer has primary coverage and has to pay the medical expenses, minus deductibles and co-insurance payments which could then be covered by Medicare, as second- ary coverage; if they are more than the current Medicare deductibles and co-payments, you should get something from Medicare, if not, I wouldn't count on much, if anything.

Medicare coverage has two parts:

Part A pays the *hospital* and/or skilled nursing facility.

Part B pays additional *medical* expenses (mostly doctors, etc.).

Part A coverage is automatic when you become entitled to Social Security benefits; Part B is optional (but the burden is on you to state that you don't want it) and currently (1991) costs $29.95 which is taken out of your Social Security check, monthly (by 1993, it is expected to be $35 a month).

PART A

The in-hospital deductible, now (1991) is for the *first* 60 days of confinement; which means that you pay the first $628 and Medicare pays the rest of what is "approved" for all covered charges (like regular health insurance – the extra charges for a private room or a private nurse, plus television rental or telephone calls are *not* covered expenses).

During the next 30 days (61st to the 90th) of confinement, Part A pays all approved amounts for covered services, except for $157 a day, which you have to pay (your co-payment).

If you stay more than 90 days, continuously (one benefit period), you may draw on your lifetime (one-time or not renewable) reserve days, of which you have a total of 60; then Part A pays the approved amounts for all covered services, except for $314 a day (which, coincidentally, is about the average cost, nationally, of a hospital room per day, nowadays).

Part A also covers a "skilled" nursing facility (if it is approved or "certified" by Medicare); if you have been in a hospital, for at least 3 *days* (consecutively, not counting the day of discharge), before entering the skilled nursing facility (SNF). The admission to the SNF should be within *30 days* of your discharge from the hospital, and it should be certified by your physician as to need and cause (in relation to the condition for which you were hospitalized). If you qualify, Medicare pays for the first *20 days*, then you pay *up to* $78.50 per day, and Medicare pays the rest (if there is any) for each day, from the 21st day to the 100th day. After the 100th day, you are on your own.

Hopefully, you can find a skilled nursing facility that charges less than $78.50 a day; if not, at least you know what the limit of your cost is (for 80 days). Again, all the (above) amounts are for 1991, and as the *Guide to Health Insurance for People with Medicare* says, "these amounts are subject to change, annually."

Note: This guide is available from insurance companies (and their agents), and the U.S. Department of Health and Human Services, 6325 Security Boulevard, Baltimore, MD 21207. It is sent automatically (and annually) to those who are covered by Medicare, or soon will be covered. You should apply for Medicare before you are 65 (64 1/2 years, or older, or if you become disabled). Check with your Social Security office, or write to the above address.

There is also Part A coverage for "home health care" which includes:
 · intermittent skilled nursing services and
 · certified physical and speech therapy.

If you are confined to your home, and under the care of a physician, Part A can also cover (reasonable and necessary expenses):
 · intermittent home health aide (part-time)
 · medical social services
 · medical supplies,
 · and a portion of the cost of durable medical equipment provided under a plan of care established and periodically reviewed by a physician.

Part A does *not* cover:
· full-time nursing care
· drugs (prescriptions)
· meals delivered to your home
· or homemaker services that are primarily to assist you in meeting personal or house-keeping needs.

Hospice care is covered for those who are certified as terminally ill, and enrolled in a Medicare-certified hospice program provided by a Medicare-certified facility. There is no deductible; but, some cost-sharing for:
· outpatient drugs, and
· inpatient respite care

ASSIGNMENT AND APPEAL

The main concern of Medicare recipients should be to establish that prospective provid-ers (hospitals, skilled nursing homes, doctors, etc.) are approved or certified by Medicare – which means that they are able and willing to accept what Medicare will pay them. The process is called "assignment." The schedule of charges is set by Medicare, and is similar to UCR which is used by Blue Cross/Shield, except that it is probably less generous.

Medicare uses DRGs (diagnosis-related groups) which Yale University devised in 1975 (and are updated, accordingly) for hospital expenses, including recommended lengths of stays for particular procedures.

PPS or prospective payment system, developed by the Health Care Finance Administration in 1983, is used to determine doctors' expenses.

So, if a hospital accepts you (and vice versa) as a Medicare patient, when you sign the admission forms, one of them is assigning your Medicare payments. The only problem is (unless you want to pay for the extra time), the DRGs for hospital stays have a reputation for being a little stingy – so, don't expect to stay a long time, or "malinger," even if you *are* an "old person."

If you have a complaint, each certified hospital is supposed to have a PRO (peer review organization – doctors examining each other's opinions) to which you can appeal. If they don't have one, or you didn't like what was determined, you can appeal to the state PRO office (their address should be given to you upon admission).

Complaints on other services covered by Part A are handled by Medicare "intermediaries." You have 60 days, if you disagree with a decision, from the time that you receive it. You can submit it to the intermediary or you can go through Social Security.

If you still disagree and the amount in question is over $100 ($200 for PRO decisions) you have another 60 days to request a hearing by an administrative law judge. Cases involving $1,000 or more ($2,000 or more for PRO cases) can even be appealed to a federal court.

Part B medical coverage is handled by "carriers." After you receive your "explanation of Medicare benefits" form which breaks down your Medicare claim (after it has been processed); you have 6 months, if you disagree with a decision (from its date) to ask the carrier to review it. Then, if you disagree with its written explanation, and the amount in question is $100 or more (over the last 6 months), you have another 6 months (from the second review date) to request a hearing before a "carrier hearing officer."

"If you disagree with the carrier hearing officer's decision and the amount in question is $500 or more, you have 60 days

from the date you receive the decision to request a hearing before an Administrative Law Judge. Cases involving $1,000 or more can eventually be appealed to a federal court."

"If you are a member of an HMO (health maintenance organization) or CMP (competitive medical plan) with a Medicare contract, decisions about coverage and payment for services will usually be made by the HMO/CMP." **The Medicare Handbook**

CMPs and HMOs also have QROs (quality review organizations) which are like PROs (peer review organizations, earlier); in fact, in about half the (United) States, they are the same organization.

PART B

Medicare Part B covers approved amounts of:

· Physicians' and surgeons' services regardless of where they are received; in the hospital or clinic, at the doctor's office, or at home
· Physical therapy, speech pathology
· X-rays and lab tests
· Certain ambulance services

· Medical supplies

· 80% of the cost of durable medical equipment: wheelchairs, walkers, etc.

· Prescriptions: Inpatient drugs have always been covered. Outpatient drugs are still being debated in Congress – like catastrophic care (for 1989) was repealed, they may be a victim of the "economy."

The 1991 Part B deductible is *$100* (which is what you pay on the first $100 of medical expenses for the calendar year); after that Medicare pays 80% and you pay 20% of the "approved amounts" for covered services that are received during the rest of the year. You pay 100% of the amounts that are above the approved charges.

Medicare ends up paying (bottom line) about *half or more* of the typical medical expense.

Example: $1,000 outpatient surgery. Medicare might approve $800 (maybe less); this means that you must pay the first $100 (the deductible, unless satisfied during the calendar year), then Medicare pays 80% of the next $700 or *$560*. You owe the balance of the 20% of $700 or $140, plus the $200 that was over the approved amount, plus the $100 deductible; for a total of *$440*.

78

Another example; Part A coverage: A hospital stay of 5 days (the average is about a week) at a cost of $1500, or $300 a day (about the national average). You pay $682 (the initial hospital deductible), and Medicare pays $818 (the balance). Medicare gets better when you stay longer (if you can), at least for the first 60 days. Part B would cover the *medical* expenses as in the previous example.

EXCLUSIONS:

Expenses *not* covered by Medicare:
· Private duty nursing
· Custodial or intermediate nursing home care
· Care received outside of the USA (except some, in Canada and Mexico)
· Dental care or dentures
· Eye or ear exams, eyeglasses or hearing aids
· Cosmetic surgery (elective)
· Routine physicals or foot care and immunizations
· The first 3 pints of blood (unless replaced by donation)

There is some duplication in Medicare coverage, between Parts A and B, and some confusion about medical expenses and supplies (durable medical equipment, etc.). Basically, Part A pays *hospital* costs (like Blue *Cross*), and Part B covers *medical* expenses (like Blue *Shield*) (see Chapter 1). Home health care services are covered by both (in case you don't have one, or the other); or

> *"If you have both Medicare hospital insurance (Part A) and medical insurance (Part B), your hospital insurance pays for home health services. But Part B will pay for home health services if you do not have Part A." The Medicare Handbook, 1990.*

This handbook and publications in regard to: hospice benefits (513W), prepayment (HMOs and CMPs) plans (515W), second opinions (545W), employer health plans (602V), and "Medicare Coverage of Kidney Dialysis and Kidney Transplant Services" (603V) which is a supplement to the handbook; are free, and available, by mail, from the

Consumer Information Center
Department 59, Pueblo, CO 81009.

Since 1972, Medicare covers persons under age 65 who have been entitled to Social Security disability benefits for 24 months (consecutively); also, persons who need kidney dialysis or a kidney transplant because of end-stage renal disease.

Note: For 1991, Congress has added mammogram screening as a covered benefit; and has placed a limitation on balance billing of 125% of the Medicare approved physician's charge, with a further limit of 115% in 1992.

Also, if you don't know – Medicare providers (including doctors), since September, 1990, *must* submit their claims for services rendered to Medicare *for* you (themselves).

MEDICARE SUPPLEMENTS (OR MEDIGAP) COVERAGE

Do you really need a Medicare supplement?

The average premium (annual) for a Medicare supplement is around $1,000; that is, for the average age (over 65). At age 65, the premiums are lower; but, they increase with age (on policies through insurance companies). Some are age-bracketed; for instance, the same entry rate applies to those aged 65-69, and then a premium step-up at aged 70-74, and then again at 75-80. Some policies are not available to those over age 80 (nursing home policies are especially hard to get – more later). These premiums will be adjusted annually by the trend (inflation in health care costs) and due to changes that are made in Medicare coverage.

There are cheaper supplements available; but they are limited in what they cover. To pay $1,000 a year for a supplement that pays the Part A and Part B deductible ($682 + 100) and the medical co-payment which is 20% of approved charges doesn't make sense, unless you are hospitalized at least once a year or have a serious operation. The policies that make sense, especially today (since catastrophic coverage repeal) are the ones that go beyond Medicare coverage (not just supplement it).

It is appealing to have 100% coverage for whatever the doctor charges (especially on high-cost surgery) beyond the Medicare approved amount, which is the "sizzle" some policies sell; but, it could be more important (possible cost-wise) to have extended (beyond Medicare) skilled nursing facility coverage.

Prepayment plans (HMOs and CMPs) offer Medigap coverage, which fills the gaps in the Medicare coverage, and usually is not age-bracketed, or increased automatically with age; but, that's all it usually does, cover the (gaps) deductibles and co-payments.

Somebody could write a book (or several volumes) about Medicare supplements, and if you read it, you would probably come to the conclusion that "you get what you pay for." My philosophy is, as it is with (under age 65) health insurance, that you use what money you can afford, to protect what assets that you have. It would be better to pay the Medicare deductibles ($782) yourself, if you have to, and have coverage for the possible thousands, or tens of thousands of dollars that you could incur in a nursing home.

Now, you don't have to run out and buy a nursing home policy which pays so much a day, for so many years, for a lot of premium; because there are good Medicare supplements that include extended nursing home coverage – again, make sure it's an approved "skilled nursing facility," if and when the need arises. In other words, the *gaps* in Medicare coverage aren't as important as the open-ends, which can be more expensive in the long run.

I don't know Ed McMahon personally (a handwriting analyzer said he was a nice guy) and I don't want to demean television (I watch it myself – in fact, that's where I saw the hand-writing analyzer); but, it's not a good place to buy health insurance from, especially a Medicare supplement. For whatever amount that you have to spend, you want to maximize its potential for protecting whatever you have left. I think Ed should have enough money by now; and if not, he shouldn't be taking commissions away from agents who earn their money by explaining coverages, and tailoring policies to fit their clients' needs and wants.

I don't want to pick on Ed, either; but, you shouldn't buy something because you like somebody or because of their celebrity status. You should buy it because its good for you and your situation; and, if an agent can't get you to understand or appreciate that, then you shouldn't buy from him/her either. The insurance companies that advertise on television pay stars and others, instead of agents. In fact, they might even save money, or make more money, by paying one star a lot of it, instead of paying a lot of agents a little commission. The problem is that not all coverage is the same, although some policies are similar, and you should know the difference(s); and, I don't think, even a star, can explain that, in a minute or so commercial (no matter how many times that you see it) on television.

So, don't be afraid of the deductibles. Some policies have good coverage with or without covering the deductibles – weigh the difference in premium. If you don't go into the hospital, you save money in premium. If you do go into the hospital, you have the money that you saved (if you didn't spend it). I have seen annual premiums to cover the Part B deductible that are actually more than the Medicare deductible ($100, 1991) which is annual. The reason for this is the cost of handling small claims, or at least, it should be. You are paying for paperwork, not insurance.

NURSING HOME POLICIES
(LONG TERM CARE)

Nursing home coverage is *really* a situation of paying for what you get. In most policies, you can pick out how much a day that you would want the policy to pay (from $10-100 per day, usually) and how long you would want it to pay (from 1-5 years, usually). You can also choose the waiting or elimination period which means when you would want the coverage to start. It normally starts "immediately" (from the first day that you are confined in the nursing home) *or* after the 20th day that you are confined (which is when the Medicare co-payment starts, at $78.50 a day that you pay), *or* after the 100th day (which is when the Medicare co-payment stops, and then you pay everything.

Of course, the longer that the waiting period is, the lower that the premium will be – it's like a deductible, in a way. Also, the lower that the per day benefit is, or the shorter that the length of time in the benefit period (number of years) is, the lower the premium will be (I know, it figures).

If you can't find a good Medicare supplement with any (or enough) nursing home coverage for your own peace of mind, and you want to cover this possible expense ($2-3,000 a month, for who knows how long) take a look at some nursing home, or "long term care" policies. One of the major differences in premiums (other than the above choices) will be whether you have to have previous hospitalization (usually 3 days) and then be admitted to the nursing home (usually within 14 days from the discharge date from the hospital). Some policies require this prior hospitalization, and a related cause, like Medicare does, but, note the difference – Medicare gives you *30* days (or maybe more), not *14*.

Most policies require a physician's certification of the necessity of nursing home care, and I would be suspicious of one that didn't. Also, a policy that does not require hospitalization will be more expensive, maybe twice as much as the one that does require it, every other benefit being equal. Other than the per day amounts, the benefit period, and the waiting period, this can be your most difficult and possibly most expensive decision.

The only advice that I can give in this situation, is pretty much the same as I gave in Chapter 4, **Buying Health Insurance**: Insure yourself for possible large expenses that you can't afford, and don't want to pay for with the family jewels (if there are any). In this case, it is nice to have 1st day coverage of $100 per day for 5 years with no prior hospitalization; but, when you see the premium, you'll start thinking about alternatives.

The problem is choosing between the benefits; the daily amount should depend on where you would likely be confined (not that you would like it), and how expensive is a particular nursing home, or homes in the general area? The benefit period (length of stay – check if it's cumulative or lifetime versus reinstating) depends on how tough you are, or the longevity factor in your family, and if it would be your last place of refuge.

The waiting period, in my opinion, is the easiest thing to expand, and therefore decrease the premium. As long as you go to a "skilled nursing facility," and it is approved by Medicare (prior hospitalization, and so forth), you don't need coverage for the first 20 days.

The next 80 days (at $78.50 a day, your cost) are debatable; it's your budget. I would recommend taking the longest waiting period that you can stand (financially) versus, for example, shortening the benefit period; because you have a good idea of what that will cost, and the other is open-ended.

For example: It may be better to have $40 a day, for 4 years, with a 100-day waiting period, than to have $40 a day for 3 years, with a 20-day waiting period, for about the same premium.

By the way, premiums are based on age (the younger you are, the lower the premium) and typically run from age 50 (the earliest you can apply) to age 79 (age 80, and over, is usually too old to apply). You don't have to be over 65 (unless stated) to collect, if you are confined to a nursing home. You *will* have to fill out an application to apply for a policy, and answer health questions. Generally, long-term

care is harder to get than a Medicare supplement; but shouldn't be as hard to get as (under
age 65) health insurance.

The advantage of a nursing home policy
(versus a Medicare supplement that has extended "skilled nursing facility" coverage) is
that you don't have to go to a Medicare-certified facility – most policies are very liberal in
their definition of a "nursing home;" and some
cover custodial or intermediate care, also.
These are things that you want to check in the
policy that you are looking at, and before that,
check with Medicare, or whoever, to find out if
there are "approved" (Medicare-certified)
skilled nursing facilities in you area, or an area
where you might be confined (admitted).

Another nice thing about a lot of "long
term care" policies is that they offer home
health care, as a covered expensive, as an
alternative to nursing home care. If you are
only interested in home health care, *period*;
there are also policies that are available (lately)
that specialize in just home health care coverage, and are cheaper than those that cover both
nursing home *and* home (in yours or somebody
else's home) health care.

Note: There is another waiting period that you should be aware of, and that is the one for "pre-existing conditions." A fair amount of time for this is 60 days. In other words, anything (condition) that was treated *before* the policy became effective (say, 6 months prior – 12 months is asking a lot for old folks; especially when "treatment" means taking medicine, or even getting advice), would not be covered until 60 days *after* the effective date.

If there is no waiting period for pre-existing conditions; that is, everything that everybody has is covered right away, I would be suspicious, unless the policy is very expensive. In fact, if it isn't expensive now, it will be in the near future; if it still exists.

This is really an "elimination" period, in the sense that it eliminates (by condition) the people who wait until they are ready to be admitted, and want to buy an "insurance" policy on the way in.

The idea of insurance is to cover a possible risk, not a probable event. If insurance companies' agents sold policies at the entrances of hospitals, nursing homes, etc., the premiums would amount to the cost of the stay, plus administrative (handling) charges.

MEDICAID

If the worst (in one way) happens and you outlive your policy (or if you can't afford one in the first place), and you are in a nursing home – there is help available. Medicaid will pay for a skilled nursing facility, once your own assets are depleted, at least to the poverty level. This level is around $6,000 for an individual, and around $8,000 for a married couple; the maximum income level will vary by state. Also, the amount of assets that you may have will vary, along with the time of separation from them.

In other words, if you dispose of assets (to relatives or whomever), say 2½ years before entering a nursing home, and plead poverty when you get there, those assets may not count. This is very tricky territory and I am not recommending a way to outwit the government, nor am I trying to give advice which you should seek from an attorney. Also, these laws will vary widely among states.

Medi*caid* also covers impoverished people under age 65 (and not disabled) who are not eligible for Medi*care*. The same poverty level (above) applies, although the amount of assets that you may have will also vary by state. The best thing to do, if you don't have health insurance, is to check with your Social Security or welfare office. If you qualify for Medicaid, you will receive a card that will entitle you to health care benefits, in fact, usually without deductibles or co-insurance (including prescriptions, maybe).

The problem is that not all doctors, sometimes hospitals and clinics, want to take Medicaid patients – some say it's the paperwork; but, just like with Medicare, the government is scaling down assignment amounts, and providers don't see much of a chance in getting the difference (from what they actually charge) from Medicaid recipients who are poor enough to qualify for Medicaid, in the first place.

See *SUGGESTED READING*

CHAPTER 9 – TRENDS, TAXES AND TRIVIA

The main or primary trend in health care is that of increasing costs. Without getting statistical, health care costs have outpaced inflation in general–the average costs of other goods and services–by several fold, especially since the 1950's. Some statistical caricatures that have been done for certain time-periods are mind-boggling. We all know what has happened, either at our own expense, or because of the complaints of an employer.

Pleas for National Health Insurance are being heard, not only for those who are uninsured, but for the relief of the financial pressure being put on those who have to pay premiums. We *all* pay for health insurance, either directly or indirectly. The idea behind a government plan is that a centralized authority could control costs; that is, payments to providers. I don't know of anything that has gone through Washington and come out any cheaper; in fact, most things ($700 airplane toilet seats, etc.) seem to get more expensive–ridiculously and unbelievably expensive.

One of the problems, and causes, of increasing costs (other than the binge of new and more expensive technology and equipment) is "provider greed". Doctors, and hospitals which pay doctors and others, have used their unique position in the balance of things (life, health, death) to exploit an ignorant public: not just ignorant about the marvels and mysteries of medical practice; but, also of the knowledge that would enable patients to become more critical, and therefore increase their willingness to criticize. Who is willing to criticize providers when your life is in their hands?

Physicians feel that they earn their money–whatever amount it is–because of their rigorous and lengthy education (and its costs) that is necessary to create their expertise which they say has improved over the centuries. They also distance themselves from their patients; especially surgeons, assistants, anesthetists, etc., who do not have direct contact with conscious consumers or avail themselves to criticism, or comparisons in costs. Since doctors have stopped making house calls, going to their offices and seeing their staffs has depersonalized their service and distanced them in another way. Incorporating and using impersonal billing and collection services further removes the doctor from the patient.

Specialization of physicians' services, especially surgery, has led to higher and more spread-out costs–and to more distancing. I'm not saying that this, in itself, is good or bad; but, it tends to depersonalize the patient, again. In this case, he or she is viewed in less than a holistically human way as a specific organ, or part. The "specialist" label itself vaingloriously justifies higher charges on an egotistical level, also.

Fear (out of ignorance, and of the unknown) is exploited in medicine. It probably always has been; but, because of insurance coverage, it has never had the financing that it enjoys today. Also, because the employer or the "company" usually pays for health insurance, the patient is less critical because he/she is not directly paying for it and is removed financially–in fact, most non-premium-paying patients tend to over-use the system, especially when they have the attitude that its benefits are things that they have coming to them, and they want the best of everything. They want to fly first-class, drink champagne, etc.

The underlying problem to the modern situation is that people don't want to suffer as much as they did in the past, or at least they don't seem to be as willing to, or aren't as tough about it. When legal drugs are selling in the billions of dollars a year ($6 billion plus in the U.S., and growing) it's an indication of a pain-escaping mindset. The epidemic use of illegal drugs reinforces this attitude of escapism.

When people are afraid and uncritical, they tend to be victimized individually, and enough of them have been victimized to create a problem, collectively. This weakness has given even more power to the medical community.

Another factor in the rising costs of health care is malpractice insurance. As juries and judges award more money in malpractice suits, the providers (doctors, hospitals, etc.) have to pay more in premiums for their malpractice insurance. The lawyers are kept busy and benefit from their contingency fees, but the higher premium costs are passed on to the consumers of the providers' services. As they charge more, of course, health insurance premiums rise accordingly.

The trend here seems to be reversing, or at least lessening, as far as awards are going. The age of consumerism, which has encouraged high awards, is giving way to the practicality that, although some consumers may receive large rewards, the rest of us have to pay for them. I have noticed that some state laws have changed in favor of providers (not just in medical professions) of goods and services, and are limiting the tide of award-mania.

More responsibility is being placed on the shoulders of the consumers. Hopefully, this will result in a decrease in the activity that causes suits in the first place. At least, it should create the attitude that consumers should be more careful, if not more critical, in their consuming. The idea that just because a person has insurance, he/she can act irresponsibly and the insurance company will pay for the damages, has helped to further increase costs, and premiums.

Government legislation has played a dramatic role in the spiraling costs of health care, especially Medicare/Medicaid. Now that action is being taken (DRGs and PPSs) to control or lower costs, and to correct abuses by providers, this trend will hopefully benefit the entire system, although it may increase the complaints of Medicare beneficiaries and Medicaid recipients.

COBRA has increased premiums in general, because carriers can't average risks when employees leave their group plans. Most employees who want to continue their coverage have a reason to do so–usually what would be considered a "pre-existing condition" if they tried to get new coverage, especially an individual policy. This adverse selection is the reason that conversion policies (from a group plan to an individual employee or his/her family) cost more and cover less than the preceding or former group plan.

State governments have forced insurance companies selling health insurance in their states to include certain amounts of maternity, psychiatric care, substance abuse programs, etc., coverage. Sometimes, coverage is based on a certain level or number of employees. Sometimes it is mandated; for example: covering single employees, or dependents of employees (other than spouses) for maternity expenses.

Another important trend is the placing of more direct responsibility on employees–not only to submit claims, but to pre-certify surgery (and get second opinions) and hospital stays (and stay the recommended days). Also, more companies are demanding some, or more, of a contribution toward premiums, as they continue to rise. Higher deductibles and co-payments are ways of relieving employer costs, and they also make the consuming employee more involved, and hopefully more critical.

The trend in coverage is for less frills, whether they had been mandated by a state, or just unwanted because of the extra premium-cost. For example, psychiatric coverage has been diminished, if not removed; counseling services are also targets of belt-tighteners. Even the carry-over provision for calendar year deductibles has been targeted in an effort to reduce premiums.

One of the most interesting trends is in some individual and small group plans. The new policies are being touted as saving 30-35% versus major medical plans: and what are they? They are "in-hospital" policies that are basic hospital-surgical plans (usually with limited benefit periods– prior to, during and after hospitalization), that don't cover doctors' office visits, prescriptions, etc., during the rest of the year (while not in the hospital). They make sense, except for outpatient treatments such as for cancer, kidney dialysis, etc., and of course, for other outpatient services such as CAT scans (about $1,000 a shot) and MRIs, etc., which can add up fast.

Actually, the policies have come almost full-circle, back to basic Blue Cross/Shield of the 1930's/40's before major medical coverage. (see Chapter 1).

FEDERAL TAXES

If you are incorporated, of course, you can write off health insurance premiums as a business expense. The enforcement of Section 89 hasn't worked out too well; but, if you reimburse executive or key employees for their out-of-pocket (health care) expenses, you could still have a problem in writing that off as a bonus, etc. Congress is constantly looking for more money to spend, and will probably be back with another tax attack; they don't seem to be happy enough just taxing the employee for the additional income.

My best overall advice is "don't discriminate inside classes". You can define the classes (like you can with group life insurance) and the benefits can differ between them, but not within them. I'm not a tax person, but I know the IRS doesn't like discrimination!

If you are self-employed (and not incorporated, or own more than 2% of a Subchapter "S" corporation), as a sole proprietor (or partner) you can deduct 25% of what you spent in premiums for health insurance on your federal income tax form 1040 (line 26), "self-employed health insurance deduction", as an adjustment to income. This big break has been extended, again (from October 1, 1990), to January 1, 1992. It applies to premium paid for you and your eligible dependents.

If you are self-employed and have employees that are considered "full-time" and you want to take the above deduction for yourself/family, you are also supposed to pay for the employees' health insurance (or contribute at least 50% of their premium). The amount that you contribute should be treated as a business expense (Schedule C). In other words, you are not supposed to deduct your premiums unless you provide coverage for your employees, if they are eligible. This is an old IRS rule to get small businesses to cover their employees; but, like Section 89, it hasn't worked out too well, either.

If you are employed, but pay for your own health insurance, you are entitled to a deduction of the premium(s) that you have paid, subject to the 7.5% limit (long form). This means you must subtract 7.5% of your adjusted gross income from your medical expenses, which includes expenses *not* paid by your health insurance, to figure your medical expense deduction. For more information, send for IRS Publications No. 502 and No. 535 from one of the following addresses:

Forms Distribution Center
1. Rancho Cordova, CA 95743-0001
2. P.O. Box 9903, Bloomington, IL 61799
3. P.O. Box 25866, Richmond, VA 23289

(Pick the one closest to where you live, or call 1-800-829-3676. Either way, it's free.)

STATE TAXES

A few states have discussed offering relief to small businesses for the cost of health insurance by the way of state tax deductions. In fact, the new governor of Ohio, George Voinovich, may become a pioneer in this area. He has suggested in his response to the health care issue, while running for office, that Ohio should give small businesses, or all businesses that buy health insurance for their employees, a deduction on their state income taxes. This would be an incentive to those who are not currently providing this benefit, to do so; and, for those who have been, to continue doing so.

This proposal would apply mainly to small businesses (less than 20-25 employees), which is where they say that the majority of the 37 million working people and their dependents (nationally) who don't have health insurance benefits are. Of course, it probably wouldn't get through the legislative process, because it makes too much sense, and it would help cure a problem that would lessen the need for a universal health insurance plan. It would also relieve some pressure on the state's Medicaid grant money.

Governor Voinovich's proposal was in response to former Governor Dick Celeste's endorsement of an 8% payroll tax, plus some other taxes to fund a mandatory state-wide, Canadian-type (universal) plan. It would be interesting to see how one state–"the heart of it all"–could implement such an isolated adventure. By the way, in

Canada, it has been said that there are long waiting lists for certain surgeries, especially for heart surgery; and that Canadians come to the States for them, many to Ohio's Cleveland Clinic, rather than waiting in Canada.

The 8% payroll tax plan is coming up again this year, except that it now wants to impose a 9% payroll tax on employers, a 1.25% payroll tax on employees, a 10% tax on the self-employed, an excise (sin) tax on alcohol and tobacco, and a payroll surcharge tax (4.24%) to pay health costs for retirees.

State Representative Robert Hagan, D-Youngstown, is sponsoring this legislation in order to establish the "Ohio Universal Health Insurance Plan". It would create a 19-member board of governors, and the tax money would go to the "Ohio Health Care Trust Fund", which would pay the providers (doctors, hospitals, etc.) directly, "and eliminate the need for patients to fill out paperwork." *(Associated Press, 2/19/91)*

Rep. Hagan goes on to say that Canada's state-financed health care system has helped to reduce that country's infant mortality rate, and to establish a life expectancy two years longer than that in the United States. He also said, "There is always over-utilization in the beginning of any of these systems...It's something we should look out for."

Supporters say that the plan would not cost more than the $27.5 billion now spent annually on health care in Ohio. It reminds me of when the

federal income tax was started and the guy (sup-
posedly) said, "If we let 'em have 1% now, pretty
soon it will be 5%....."

TRIVIA

In New York (a state that is tough on insurance
companies) where two of three health (group)
insurance plans require employee contributions,
the cost of medical care is rising by an average of
21% a year–reports the Wyatt Co., a Washington,
D.C. benefits consulting firm. Current employee
contributions are $384 (individual) and $1,044
(family) per year, average. Deductibles have risen
to $165 (individual) and $425 (family), and out-of-
pocket limits (deductible plus co-payment) are
now $1,400 (individual) and $2,160 (family). Co-
payments are still 80% (insurer) and 20% (employee or dependent). *(UPI–1/13/91)*

Also, in Albany, N.Y.–"The state's highest court
has opened the way for health insurers to test
applicants for the AIDS virus–and deny coverage
to those who test positive. By striking down a rule
set in 1987 by the state's former superintendent of
insurance. The State Court of Appeals unani-
mously affirmed a decision made in February
(1991) by the Appellate Division of the State
Supreme Court in Albany, striking down the 1987
regulation. The February ruling held that former
State Superintendent of Insurance, James Corcoran,
lacked legal authority when he issued a rule
banning insurers from testing applicants for the
disease." *(Record-Courier, Kent-Ravenna, OH, 2/91)*

Cleveland, Ohio – A survey of 151 Ohio employers says that health care costs increased 24.8 percent last year (1990), while a related national survey showed average employee medical expenses rose 21.6 percent, nationally. According to A. Foster Higgins and Co., an employee benefits consulting firm, average Ohio medical plan costs increased from $2,638 (1989) to $3,292 (1990). Nationally, the average increased from $2,600 (1989) to $3,161 (1990), based on 1,955 employers surveyed... In Cleveland, the average cost was up 22.4 percent, from $2,779 (1989) to $3,401 (1990), according to a survey of 40 (local) employers...

"The survey showed that 99 percent of the employers responding ranked medical cost containment as the no. 1 health benefit issue facing them in the next three years. Ninety-four percent said sharing such increased costs with employees would be a part of their corporate strategy. *(Associated Press 1/31/91)*

In Columbus, Ohio (the state capital) State Rep. Paul Jones recently introduced House Bill 169, designed to provide children with better access to health care in Ohio, by mandating insurance companies to provide preventive child health care coverage. He said, "...very few insurance plans cover immunizations and other preventative services crucial to a child's development and growth...".

Last year, Jones enacted legislation establishing the Hospital Care Assurance Program, which brought $32 million in Federal money to help ensure health care access for 1.5 million uninsured Ohioans. Jones said, "In passing House Bill 738, I knew this was only the first step in solving Ohio's uncompensated care crisis. We must remember that a journey of a thousand miles must begin with one step. Well Baby Care will ensure that children receive continuous primary care, helping to reduce the incidence of more serious illness later in life..." *(Record-Courier, 3/13/91)*

In Oregon–"The leaders of the Beaver State are laying down a table of priorities for health care for the poor, taking into consideration costs and benefits. The result is a table ranking 808 medical conditions according to the cost-effectiveness of medical treatment for them. The available money (now $350 million a year for 190,000 on Medicaid) will be spent on all of the state's medically indigent people for those procedures most likely to provide the most benefit for the buck.

"For instance, huge sums will not be spent on babies of extremely low birth weight... if spending such money could deny treatment to poor patients with pneumonia, tuberculosis, peritonitis or other disorders that can be treated at relatively low cost with high expectations of full recovery." *(Record-Courier editorial, 3/14/91)*

Cleveland, Ohio–Fifty-six percent of Northeast Ohioans are willing to pay more in sin taxes (on alcohol and tobacco) and increased fines for speeding and drunken driving, to make sure that everyone (in Ohio) gets medical care–according to a Gallup poll of 501 randomly selected Ohio residents, commissioned by the Ohio and Greater Cleveland Hospital Associations.

"The majority opposed increased sales or income taxes... Nearly a third of the respondents blamed high medical costs on physicians , and 22% said hospitals contributed most significantly to rising costs...

"The hospitals are concerned about the growing number of uninsured patients, because so many of them don't pay their hospital bills. Last year, Cleveland-area hospitals provided an estimated $150 million worth of uncompensated care.

"Greater Cleveland Hospital Association officials said the poll was commissioned to gauge attitudes about health care. They declined to say how much they paid for it. Neither the Cleveland nor the Ohio Hospital Association has taken a stand on a bill that would make the state the sole insurer of all Ohioans." (Hagan's Canadian-type plan) The poll also showed that:

• 42% of respondents believe health care services are not available to people who can't afford them.

• 78% said their local hospitals provided good or excellent care.

• 79% rated the "caring and concern" at their local hospitals as good or excellent. (Doug Lefton, The Plain Dealer, 3/14/91)

Akron, Ohio – "What started out as a routine visit to the dentist escalated into a medical nightmare for a 10-year-old Akron boy..." The boy's parents allege that after a routine visit for teeth cleaning, a series of complications developed that caused massive brain damage, heart disease, partial paralysis and other problems that have ruined the boy's life.

They also claim that a local hospital mishandled the treatment of the complications and sought damages from them, too: According to sources "close to the case", a settlement in excess of $1 million was reached with the hospital.

The dentist (who the parents allege should have known) didn't give the boy (who has a congenital heart problem which could be aggravated by infection) antibiotics to prevent an infection from bleeding (from the cleaning). The boy got bacterial endocarditis which was misdiagnosed by local doctors as viral flu. He eventually worsened until he required two emergency brain operations to stop its bleeding.

"Since then the boy has required more than $200,000 in medical care, including 2 heart valve replacements, and he will require more expensive treatment in the future, the family says." The dentist and doctors are involved in a malpractice suit which was filed by the parents, and is going to trial this. (The original teeth-cleaning was in June, 1986). *(Jim Quinn, Beacon Journal, 4/8/91)*

Ravenna, Ohio – Employees (members of the United Rubber Workers) at a local manufacturer are striking over company attempts to pass on higher health insurance costs to them. Union officials said that the company had made a good offer, but refused to honor a union demand to set a limit on health insurance premiums.

The employees' first contributions (in 1988) were: $12 (single), $21 (two-person), and $30 (family) per month. As of January, 1991 they are: $20 (single), $35 (two-person), and $46 (family) per month. The company (under a self-insured plan) has also been increasing deductibles and co-payments... *(Record-Courier, 4/3/91)*

New York – Under the "Business Mirror" column, the heading "No Quick Answers to High Health Care Costs" begins an article which is a tirade of frustration in regard to the health care problem. It ends with:
"...Statistics document the ominous move toward some kind of ultimatum.

• Health-care expenditures last year rose to 12.2 percent of the gross national product.

• Government at all levels spent nearly 15 percent of revenue on health care in 1989. In 1965, the comparable figure was 5 percent.

• Health care expenditures have grown faster than the gross national product in all but three years since 1960.

In 1989...health-care spending exceeded $604 billion..." *(Associated Press, 5/5/91)*

In 1991, health-care spending is expected to exceed $650 billion, or about 12% of the GNP.

Chapter 10 – Dental, Disability, etc...

This is the most difficult chapter for me, because it is the last one, and I can't get excited about the subjects (which is why I put them together, and saved them). Dental plans are pretty much superfluous to health insurance, and disability plans (because of Workers' Compensation and Social Security) are another luxury–although a lot of people might not agree with me.

A dental plan can be a good deal when the company (if it's a corporation) provides it as an incentive to new (prospective) employees, and as a morale builder for current employees, because the company can write it off as a business expense. If you have to pay for a dental plan, you would be better off (there are exceptions–who raise the premiums) paying the dentist yourself. Most small-group plans don't have very extensive coverage, as some want to believe–especially orthodontic coverage (for straightening teeth) is limited, if it is even included.

Like everything else (for example, an indemnity policy which pays so much a day for a hospital room, and so much for surgery) you get what you pay for, minus the costs of claims-handling and administration. I'm not trying to put these processors out of work; but, that's what it boils down to, bottom line.

There is no great (financial) risk involved in dental coverage. Gum disease, TMJ (jaw disorder–see appendix) and other expensive problems probably won't be covered anyhow. It may seem convenient to have someone else pay the dentist (especially if his/her office fills out the forms and submits them for you); but, it costs.

All that dental plans have done to the health insurance market, other than providing a little commission to agents, is to raise the price of dental services. Maybe more people have gone to the dentist because of this benefit, and have cleaner teeth, and hopefully a healthier mouth; but it's hard to appreciate that as a social development, unless they have made the air cleaner and easier to breathe (at least for those around them).

If you must buy a dental plan, the most important thing to consider is the schedule, and then the percentage (or part) of the scheduled amount that the plan will pay. Most dental plans have waiting periods, especially for certain (more expensive) procedures. In most group plans the carriers demand total participation of the employees (eligible, by their definition). The only exception would be spousal coverage in another dental plan; even if an employee doesn't have any teeth!. Late entrants (not enrolling upon employment) can be treated as severely as with health insurance. (see Chapter 7).

110

A sample of dental coverage (although it is not typical) is a plan that is marketed by a Cleveland-area insurer as a part of a so-called group (one employee is enough–there is a monthly administrative fee, like most dental plans) health insurance trust:

The first year, the plan pays 20%.

The second year it pays 40%.

The third year it pays 60%.

The fourth year it pays 80%.

The fifth year and thereafter, it pays 100 percent of the schedule (not what the dentist charges). What the agents fail to tell their clients (who become members of this trust), or what the clients fail to remember (at least the ones with whom I have talked) is that for the year(s) to count, you have to have an exam, cleaning, etc., during that year (and consecutively, without missing a year), or you remain at, or go back to, 20 %.

A man I met told me this story of how he had waited 5 years, gone to the dentist, had his exam, teeth cleaned, etc., and then submitted his claim (thinking that he would be reimbursed for the bill that he had paid). This was a few years ago, and the bill was only $30.00 (he evidently didn't need any fillings); but, when he opened the statement from the insurance company, the enclosed check was for $1.40.

He said that he didn't know that he had to go to the dentist every year (or that there was a schedule), so he only received 20%. The schedule at that time–(based on when he started the plan) paid $7.00 for the service(s): so, 20% of the $7.00 equals $1.40. It's a true story.

DISABILITY INCOME

If everyone were honest, and had to pay a premium to a disability plan, it would be like Workers' Compensation. If there were no arsons, fire insurance would be a fraction of what it costs. Insurance companies act like the police department, in this case, making an attempt to catch the (criminals) fraudulent claims-makers. But if they were to really do their job and get rid of them (put them all in jail), then they would both be out of business.

Because it will probably take up to a year and a half to get Social Security benefits for a bona-fide disability, short-term disability income is a legitimate benefit. Depending on how good or bad your state's Workers' Compensation program is, basically, the idea of disability income is sold as a supplement to state and/or federal benefits which may be less than you are accustomed to, and slow in coming (at least in the beginning).

Most long term disability income plans pay up to age 65, or a bit longer, and have elimination periods as long as short term coverage (1-2 years) is, altogether.

Group plans, like dental plans, offer better coverage (as a rule); but, companies (especially, large ones) tend to decrease benefits over time, to lower premiums. Although disability rates have been very stable, (they are basically indemnity policies for specific amounts), they have suffered under the crunch of increases in health care costs and premiums.

Individual policies (and small group, usually less than 10 employees) are very much like long-term care policies. You choose the benefit period (the length of time that you want to be compensated), the elimination period (after which the payments will start), and the amount that you want to receive (usually monthly, and subject to a percentage of your working income).

Short-term disability is good coverage for the time that it takes to get Social Security (12 months of disability, then 5+ months of processing). It is especially good if you are self-employed and/or not covered by Workers' Compensation. The elimination period is usually 1 day for accidents, and 7 or 8 days for sickness (as the cause of disability). These periods can be increased in order to lower premiums (which are not cheap). In some (less desirable) occupations or professions, if disability coverage is even offered, the insurer will automatically impose longer elimination periods. Disability carriers can be very picky.

The payment (benefit) amount varies between less than 50% and up to 70% (possibly, a little more), and is usually 60% or 66 % of provable income. If you are self-employed, you will have to show a believable income stream, not just a cash flow, for a significant period of time (history). If you go with a plan that pays a percentage (not a specific amount), find out if it is based on gross, adjusted, net or "whatever" income, and if that income is what you were earning when (if) you become disabled. These percentage-type policies usually offer an "inflation-guard", which means that the benefit amount will increase with time (which is what your income is supposed to do) and, of course, so will your premiums.

The definition of "disability" in the policy language is probably the most important print that you want to understand. Some policies want you to become completely disabled (not able to do *any* work) while most others only require that you are unable to work at your specific trade, occupation, etc.. The latter ones, of course, are more expensive, because more claims will be paid on the more lenient definition.

To compute what you will need in the form of income (if you decide that you want disability coverage), you need to figure out what your liabilities (monthly payments, etc.) are, and how long and how much you would receive from Social Security and/or Workers' Compensation. This information is available from their offices.

If you are really interested, try to find a good agent that specializes in, or at least understands, disability coverage. (He/she will be harder to find than a good health insurance agent–or could be one in disguise.) In general, life insurance agents would be the next likeliest to know anything about disability (disability comes under the health/life license–casualty is usually a different license, test, etc., although they may be combined in some states). Casualty (home, auto, etc.) agents would be the least likely to help you. (See the end of Chapter 5–Whom To Buy From.)

DREADED DISEASE COVERAGE

Cancer is, by far, the most popular of the "dreaded diseases" that these policies (almost always individual) are designed to cover. Sometimes, an insurance company will offer a rider for cancer (or Alzheimer's disease, for example, on a Long Term Care policy); if it does, the policy itself must be suspect. Even for cancer, a rider shouldn't be necessary, if it's a good policy.

The same thing is true, if you are considering a separate cancer policy–if you need it because of inadequate coverage on your existing policy–you might need a new policy altogether (in the first place). If it doesn't cover cancer (and its possible expenses), what else could happen that wouldn't be covered?

Today, everything in medical care is expensive, and because of complications, and the availability of other diseases, separate policies aren't really the answer. They are also, by nature, "iffy" propositions. Being specific in coverage, there is more room for exceptions; automatic waiting or elimination periods; pre-existing conditions from parents (dead or alive); stipulations, such as being hospitalized for a certain time-period to qualify for benefits, waiting periods between confinements, and so on... Usually these policies are limited to small, specific amounts for hospital/surgical costs, which makes them attractively cheap. The problem is, as with old indemnity policies, if payments are based on a hospital stay (so much a day, after so many days), more and more treatment is being done on an outpatient basis these days.

Remember, "major medical" (if it's true) covers anything that is "medically necessary" (the language should be stated in the policy or certificate, Chapter 1). It would be better to have a major medical policy (or catastrophic coverage) than to have several separate policies–even if you have to take a high deductible; at least you have an idea what your out-of-pocket expenses will be. If you have a limited plan (even a portfolio of several policies), your exposure is open-ended (beyond the limits) and unknown.

If you think that the extra money from a cancer policy will help you with your out-of-pocket expenses, maybe it would–if you got the money. What you do know is that the money you would spend on the premium (however little, if you save it) is real, and could be used the same way.

The psychological problem of specific disease policies is that by having one, you might start worrying about all the other possible diseases that exist, and never feel adequately covered. If you want peace of mind (and that's why we buy insurance), spend your money (and some time understanding where it's going), on what would be good coverage for your wants/needs. If you are not comfortable with your current policy, and/or your agent isn't helping you, there are many others out there that may be better. With the basic understanding of this book, and a little specific effort on your part, you should be able to find one, or the other, or both.

EXTRA TRIVIA

"Report Blasts Bill for State Insurance"
By Doug Lefton, Plain Dealer Reporter

"A bill that would make the state the provider of health insurance to all Ohioans would be a financial disaster, says a report to be issued today by Blue Cross and Blue Shield of Ohio.

"But State Rep. Robert R. Hagan, D-53, of Youngstown, who introduced the bill, dismissed the report's findings....

"The report says the Universal Health Insurance Plan would fall $7 billion short of meeting its costs in its first year....

"Under the plan, health insurance companies in Ohio would probably go out of business, said Stephen P. Adams, a Blue Cross spokesman....

"The study said there would be an increased use of medical services under the universal plan because everyone would have full coverage. That was a major reason revenues, which the study projected at $29 billion, would not match costs, projected at $36 billion....

"The plan would be financed by a 9% *to 13%* payroll tax on employers, depending on the size of the firm... a 1.25% income tax to be paid by employees, and a 10% sales tax on tobacco and liquor." *(Cleveland Plain Dealer, 5/91)*

Washington – The GAO (General Accounting Office) is recommending the Canadian government-run health system:

"...The short-term administrative costs savings alone are more than adequate to cover any reasonable estimate of extending health care to everyone in the United States, their report said.

"Tax savings might even be large enough to eliminate the deductibles and co-payments that Americans with medical insurance now pay, making health insurance free for everyone, said the GAO, a congressional investigative agency."

This report said the Canadian system has been "clearly better" than the U.S. system in controlling costs which have been growing at the annual average rate of 1.1% in Canada, compared with 2.5% in the U.S.

"Health-care spending is heading for a 15 percent share of the GNP by the turn of the century, experts predict... Adopting a Canadian-style would save about $67 billion in administrative costs, the GAO estimated." *Associated Press (6/4/91).*

And so it goes....

Appendix

Odds and Ends

Surgery Requiring A Second Opinion

Here is a short list (liberal);
    Cholecystectomy (gall bladder)
    Heart Surgery (anything)
    Hysterectomy (females)
    Joint Surgery (hips, etc.)
    Laminectomy (back)
    Prostate (males)

plus; here is a long list (conservative);
    Adenoidectomy
    Bladder Repair
    Breast Operations
    Bunionectomy (toes)
    Carpal Tunnel Syndrome
    Cataract Extraction (eye)
    D & C (dilation and curetage)
    Hammertoe Repair
    Hemorrhoidectomy
    Hernia Repair
    Knee Survery
    Submucous Resection (nose)
    Tonsillectomy
    Varicose Vein Removal

These are just examples and not all-inclusive. Also, carriers and reviewers differ; so, when in doubt, call first.

Questionable Surgery

Weight loss or weight loss control surgery usually isn't covered under a standard health insurance contract. Blue Cross or an HMO may be more lenient, depending on their particular situations of supply and demand. According to "major medical" coverage, it could be covered if it was "medically necessary", which your doctor may have to prove.

Cosmetic surgery (elective), especially "tummy tucks", etc., are not covered expenses; but, cosmetic surgery that becomes necessary because of an accident is covered; or as a result of an infection or disease which began while the policy was in force. Replacement and repair of teeth damaged in an accident would be covered—if caused by disease (unless it's organic), teeth would probably not be covered.

TMJ – temporomandibular joint surgery or therapy (also craniomandibular disorder) probably won't be covered, unless specified in your policy or certificate of insurance. It is usually referred to as a dental problem; but, dental plans won't cover it, either. The only real chance you have of it being covered is when the person with the disorder has been born under the plan, and the claim is made when that person is still covered under that plan. Once you change plans, the new carrier can say that it was a congenital birth defect which should have been covered under the old plan, and therefore it is a pre-existing condition.

It would be easier in a large group (true group, with a complete takeover of benefits) to have TMJ surgery or therapy covered, especially if symptoms begin under the current plan. It sounds like a simple problem, but surgery for one side of the jaw can cost $5,000, and both sides are usually recommended (to be done). New surgery, notably at Cleveland Western Reserve University, is being taught which lessens the trauma, recovery and costs. If a jaw is injured because of an accident, coverage is more likely.

Birth Defects are covered automatically by a federal mandate. This happened because companies were weasling out of this coverage in various ways. Blue Cross used to have a 4-day time limit in which they had to be notified, or the new baby wouldn't be covered *until* they received a notice, which (by that time, if it was after 4 days) ruled out birth defects, as a pre-existing condition. In other words, if they received the notice 8 days after the birth, that's when the coverage began (not at birth).

Some insurers (in the past) just wouldn't cover birth defects, period. This led to a standard of at least 30-31 days, for notice of a birth; some carriers allow more time, maybe 45, or more, days.

Note: Regardless of whether there are any obvious birth defects, notify your carrier as soon as possible, preferably (but, don't wait) with the baby's name. If you wait too long, and something that is wrong with the baby is discovered later–the baby could be treated as a "late entrant" (Chapter 7), and the birth defect regarded as a pre-existing condition.

Also, if you have a step-rated plan (versus the old-fashioned family plan) your premium will go up a little (with the new child being added)–unless you have reached your per child(ren) maximum, which is normally 3-4 children. When a child leaves the family, the premium is reduced, accordingly.

Dependent Children to be eligible for coverage are defined as "unmarried" and usually:
- under 19 years of age (sometimes 18 or 21); or
- over 18 (19-21, maybe) and under age 23 (24 or 25) and *not* employed on a full-time basis, and enrolled in an accredited school or college as a full-time student (as defined by the school or college).

Note: Coverage doesn't usually stop on the actual birthday, itself; sometimes it will stop at the end of the birthday month, the end of a payment period, or possibly the end of the birthday year (latest trend). Check your policy.

"Dependent" may *not* include: (child or spouse)
- residing out of the United States,
- in the military (of any country),
- insured as an employee.

"Child" means residing in your household, and; solely supported by you:
- a natural child,
- your step-child, or
- legally adopted child.

"Dependent Spouse" means your spouse by legal marriage.

Note: If you, as the applicant (or employee in whose name the coverage is in) die, or leave your spouse because of divorce or dissolution, your ex-spouse does not have to give evidence of insurability (good health) to maintain current coverage under your plan. This applies to employees in groups of less than 20 (not under COBRA rules), and even to those who are self-employed (or unemployed) as long as the current coverage is kept in force. The premium (except for "family plans") should be reduced by the amount that applied to the deceased, after notice is given to the insurance carrier.

Marital Counseling usually isn't covered (maybe Blue Cross), unless your doctor can get your insurer to believe that it is medically necessary–maybe to save someone's life. Go for psychiatric care. It's limited, but it usually pays about 50% of so many visits per period, if covered.

Transexual Surgery (gender change) Don't even think about it–not even with Blue Cross!

Transplants are not automatically covered, even if they are "medically necessary", although they may be open to review. There should be some special language regarding transplants in your policy (or certificate). If an operation is approved, it will probably be subject to special conditions or rules. Some plans offer a transplant rider, for a little extra premium; it still may not cover everything, especially artificial organs, or experimental procedures.

General Exclusions: (all plans)

- Care *not* prescribed by a physician or P.O.P. (professional other provider)
- Care received from a relative (near)
- Experimental or investigative services (not approved by the A.M.A.–American Medical Association)
- Drugs not approved by the F.D.A. (Food and Drug Administration)
- Travel, rest cures, massages, mineral baths, or other items of personal service.
- Charges that are covered by:
    - Workers' Compensation, or Occupational Disease Laws, etc. (work-related)
    - Veterans Administration (war-related), or any government plan
- Routine physicals, foot care, flu shots (maybe innoculations, Medicare)
- Eye, ear or dental care and exams; (unless needed because of an accident; chewing or biting doesn't count)
- Custodial care or personal hygiene services
- Self-inflicted injury or sickness; voluntary participation in a riot, as a result of illegal activity, driving while intoxicated.
- Birth control drugs. They are covered in Texas (mandated); oral contraceptives are covered by some prescription plans (Cards).
- Well baby care (unless specified, or covered by a rider)
- Routine nursery care
- Circumcision (unless the doctor is Jewish)
- In-vitro fertilization

- Artificial insemination
- Sterilization (some plans cover all costs, or a percentage)
- Elective abortion (only Blue Cross ever has)
- Acts of war, atomic explosion, and radiation sickness or disease
- Air conditioners, air purifiers, or dehumidifiers, etc.
- Hearing aids; eyeglasses, or contact lenses, etc. (unless you have vision coverage).
- Some policies automatically exclude expenses caused by named hazardous activities; such as, flying, rodeo riding, car racing, etc.
- Treatment for obesity; mainly dieting or weight loss programs
- Educational services or supplies, for vocational or training purposes
- Charges paid by a responsible third party–judgements, settlements, etc. (other insurance coverage) examples; car accident, malpractice suit, etc.
- Charges paid under a "no-fault" auto insurance plan

Partially Covered Expenses:

- Psychiatric care
- Physiotherapy

The Blues have been more liberal in these benefits, but they are clamping down. HMO/PPO coverage depends on the availability of local services. These types of benefits are usually limited to so many outpatient visits–per week, per month, and total per year–and always subject to a limited number of days of inpatient care per year. Of course, they are subject to your calendar year deductible (or a separate deductible), and the co-insurance is usually 50-50%, or less.

Most plans have a lifetime benefit for all expenses related to mental or nervous disorders, and/or substance abuse treatment combined; physical medicine and rehabilitation services may be included, or have a special limit.

Example: *"Each covered person is eligible for a maximum payment of $25,000 lifetime for all covered services for all inpatient and outpatient charges for treatment of psychiatric disorders, alcoholism and/or drug addiction; for outpatient treatment of psychiatric disorders, there is a maximum payment of $1,000 per covered person in each calendar year."*

or: *"$1,000 - outpatient psychiatric care"*
   "$1,000 - outpatient substance abuse"
   "$10,000 - inpatient psychiatric and substance abuse"
   "$10,000 - physical medicine and rehabilitation services"

Some plans may limit lifetime benefits for all of the above services to $5,000, or less, however received. Also, states may mandate certain standards, to lifetime or particular benefits.
For example;
   Ohio: Chemical dependency and mental illness
      $8,000 - lifetime (aggregate)
      $4,000 - in any 24-month period
      $1,000 - outpatient, per calendar year
      and 30 days - inpatient, per calendar year.

Chiropractic care has been covered for quite some time–if you have a very old policy, and it is not namely excluded (even though it isn't mentioned), it would probably be covered as a convention to you; but, coverage is usually limited to one visit per week, or a total of so many visits per year (20-50, normally).

Hospital Confinement Rider. Some insurance companies sell a rider (supplement) to their health insurance policies and Medicare supplements that will pay so much a day for each day that you are confined in a hospital, usually in increments of $50 a day. This is the same thing as an indemnity policy, except that it is part of another policy.

Example:

You could pay $3.50 per month at age 20, and up to $14.00 per month at age 64, and receive $50.00 a day for each day that you are confined in the hospital (because of a covered injury or illness). If you have a family that is applying for coverage, and you want the rider, all members must be included.

This rider has been a nice idea, and the money could be used to cover your deductible and/or co-payment; but, the problem (today) is that it's hard to stay very long in the hospital. Because of cost-containment and the attitude (backlash) at the hospitals, you are more likely to be sent to a nursing home (especially, if you are older, over 65) or just sent home.

Height and Weight Charts

These charts are designed (and vary) by companies. They are printed for underwriters at the home offices, and distributed (in some cases) to agents in the field, for the purpose of assessing the insurability of an applicant. I am reprinting an average of several companies' charts that I have dealt with, to give a general idea of their guidelines. Like other information in this book, it is not for the purpose of outwitting the insurance company.

Remember, if you give fraudulent information, your coverage can be nullified or voided. Beginning in 1991, Ohio has required agents to make prospective applicants of health (and life) insurance aware of this with a written notice:

"As per requirements by the State of Ohio, we are notifying you that: any person who, with intent to defraud or knowing that he (she) is facilitating a fraud against an insurer, submits an application or files a claim containing a false or deceptive statement is guilty of insurance fraud."

As I said in Chapter 3 (Buying Health Insurance), even omissions can cause problems during the contestability period (the first two years of the policy); now, you can add possible punishment.

Also, insurers can (and regularly do) want an attending physician's statement from your doctor and/or a paramedical exam (if you don't have a doctor), or if they just feel like it. One of the things that is done (routinely) in a paramedical exam is a height/weight measurement.

These charts are also used to compute a substandard surcharge which increases the premium for that particular applicant (sometimes, in a small group, it will be a percentage on the whole premium). The range from the standard height/weight figure to the non-acceptable level is usually from 15-100% (increase in premium). This would be in addition to surcharges for other conditions, so you could become uninsurable by quantity (say, a total of 100%, which is double the standard premium, for your age and sex).

If you are under/overweight maybe the chart will give you an incentive to gain/reduce, as the case may be–unless you can get taller or shorter. By the way, I feel that they are very liberal, especially versus the old Metropolitan Life table from the 1950's which was used until recently, and according to which you had to be very thin or very tall.

Also, don't be discouraged. If you are otherwise in good health, but not on the charts, it is still possible to get a health insurance policy. Usually, interim or temporary (up to 12 months) health insurance doesn't ask for your height/weight. It will give you time to gain/reduce or get shorter-taller (more later)...

Male - Weight

Height	Standard	Rated	Not Acceptable
4'10"	82-174	175-225	226+
4'11"	89-178	179-231	232+
5'0"	91-182	183-234	235+
5'1"	94-184	185-237	238+
5'2"	96-188	189-243	244+
5'3"	99-192	193-247	248+
5'4"	102-197	198-255	256+
5'5"	105-202	203-262	263+
5'6"	108-207	208-269	270+
5'7"	112-212	213-276	277+
5'8"	115-218	219-284	285+
5'9"	120-224	225-293	294+
5'10"	123-229	230-298	299+
5'11"	127-235	236-306	307+
6'0"	131-240	241-312	313+
6'1"	136-248	249-323	324+
6'2"	142-254	255-329	330+
6'3"	147-261	262-339	340+
6'4"	152-269	270-355	350+
6'5"	158-277	278-359	360+
6'6"	164-285	289-369	370+
6'7"	170-294	295-379	380+
6'8"	176-303	304-389	390+

Female - Weight

Height	Standard	Rated	Not Acceptable
4'10"	79-145	149-193	194+
4'11"	81-151	152-196	197+
5'0"	83-154	155-200	200+
5'1"	85-157	158-205	206+
5'2"	87-160	161-209	210+
5'3"	90-164	165-212	213+
5'4"	93-168	169-218	219+
5'5"	96-172	173-221	222+
5'6"	98-175	176-225	226+
5'7"	102-179	180-231	232+
5'8"	106-183	184-236	237+
5'9"	110-188	189-243	244+
5'10"	114-194	195-250	251+
5'11"	118-200	201-256	257+
6'0"	122-208	209-268	269+
6'1"	126-214	215-275	276+
6'2"	130-220	221-282	283+
6'3"	134-226	227-290	291+
6'4"	138-232	233-298	299+

Surcharge by Condition

There are so many health problems (conditions) that could require a surcharge (or possibly a rider, or both) that they are not worth listing. In general, anything (other than colds or flu) that has been treated in the past 1,2,3,4,5-10 years, depending on the severity of the disease or condition (illness or injury) can be surcharged.

The time-period of the surcharge, and the percentage of the increase in premium will be determined by how serious the condition was (or still is), and these factors:

1. The length of time since the last treatment

2. The likelihood of further expense (recurrence of the problem, or complications)

3. The number of people in your group. The underwriting is tougher, when fewer are applying, if it's a group plan. Individual policies are under-written separately, even if they are submitted together (multiple policies with one carrier).

4. The seriousness of future problems, the probability of high costs.

Declinations (turn-downs)

This list is taken from individual policy under-writing buidelines, but it will also apply to small group plans until they become large enough to be "true groups" or become eligible for a complete takeover of benefits (Chapter 4): That is, when the carrier doesn't require a health history of individual employees (applicants). Again, the more people in the group, the more willing are the underwriters to take a "ringer", although under-writing has been getting tougher over time, in general.

These conditions and diseases will likely cause an applicant to be declined. The number of years refers to the recovery period, which means no treatment (possibly, including medicine) for that length of time:

Addison's Disease
Alcoholism (5 years)
Alzheimer's Disease
Amputation (due to disease)
Amyotrophic Lateral Sclerosis
Anemia (Sickle Cell, Aplastic)
Aneuryism (6 years, maybe)
Apoplexy
Arteriosclerosis (5 years)
Brain Tumor (Malignant)
Buerger's Disease (possibly)
Cancer (internal-5 years)
Cardiovascular Renal Disease
Cerebral Palsy (possibly)
Cerebral Thrombosis
Chondromalacia
Chrone's Disease (5 years)
Chronic Pernicious Anemia
Cushing's Disease Syndrome
Cyanosis
Cystic Fibrosis (benign-5 years)
Diabetes (older onset-rider)
Diabetic Neuropathy
Down's Syndrome
Drug Abuse (5 years, maybe)
Emphysema (severe)
Heart (generally not considered;
    some conditions-5 years)
Hemiplegia, Hemophilia
Hodgkin's Disease (5 years?)
Huntington Chorea
Leukemia (5 years, maybe)
Lupus, Disseminated (systemic)

Mental Retardation
Mongoloidism
Multiple Sclerosis
Muscular Distrophy
Myasthenia Gravis
Narcolepsy (maybe 2 years)
Osteomyelitis (if disabling)
Paget's Disease, Osteitis Deformans
Paraplegia (5-10 years)
Parkinson's Disease (possibly)
Polycystic Kidney Disease
Polycythemia Vera
Polymyalgia Rheumatica
Polyneuritis
Pott's Disease
Psychoneurosis
Quadriplegia
Raynaud's Disease
Scleroderma
Syphilis, etc.
Throboangitis Obliterans
Tuberculosis (bones or joints)

This list is by no means complete, nor is it the last word. If you have (or have had) a listed condition and are otherwise in very good health, there is still hope: ultimately a decision depends on the insurance company (how hungry it is for new business); the time of their year, the time of the month, the mood of the underwriter, the phase of the moon, and many unknown factors... It's not always scientific (clear and distinct, or cut and dried).

Interim (temporary) Health Insurance can also buy some time to meet the waiting periods for certain conditions. I've been reluctant to mention interim insurance because of its temporary nature. Although most policies will continue to pay for a condition or disease that is incurred under the policy, it is limited. Also, these policies exclude pre-existing conditions altogether–back to the previous 1-5 years, or more (any treatment, including prescriptions).

I like interim because it is automatically issued (if you answer a few questions, correctly), and that eliminates underwriting hassles; but, it is only good for special situations–when a client is really clean health-wise, needs a fast-issue (usually, it is effective 12:01 a.m. of the day after the postmark), or to cover a temporary need–for example, college students on vacation (or off for a semester), or an employee between jobs (without a COBRA continuation).

Some insurers will allow you to reinstate the policy for an additional time-period. These are usually the ones that make you pay for the entire original period (up-front and non-refundable) which is usually up to 12 months (some are only 6 months, maximum). Newer policies are offering monthly payments (in advance) as you go, for 6-12 months, but without a reinstatement provision. You might be able to get another policy (with the same insurer) after a lapse; but, you will probably have to submit a new application, once.

Interim coverage is like "guaranteed issue" small group plans; but, because it's an individual policy, the pre-existing elimination period is usually longer, and there is no cash benefit allowance for pre-existing conditions (see Chapter 6). If you submit a large enough claim, though, you will probably get some underwriting, then.

Medical Information Bureau

As I mentioned in Chapter 7, insurers are using the Medical Information Bureau to obtain medical information about prospective applicants for health insurance. If you are having problems getting insurance, and feel your difficulties are unwarranted–or, you just want to know what is being reported about yourself–you have a right to this information.

M.I.B. will not give medical information directly to you, but they will furnish it to your doctor if you request it. Send your name, Social Security number, your doctor's name and address, and your signed personal request, to:

Medical Information Bureau
P.O. Box 105
Essex Station
Boston, MA 02112

Suggestions

24-Hour Coverage

If you are self-employed and not covered by a Workers' Compensation plan (it is optional in Ohio and other states–even though you have to cover employees), you want to make sure that you have "24-hour coverage" on your health insurance. Some policies (and group plans) only cover you for sickness and accidents that occur while you are *not* working. Blue Cross/Shield has especially not liked covering work-related expenses for health care; typical language to look out for, under "exclusions" is: *"Illness or injury arising out of, or in the course of employment."*

More carriers are including this coverage today (even Blue Cross is softening, because of the competition). Some companies offer it as an extra (supplemental) benefit, and will charge an extra 5-15% of your premium to include it. If you aren't covered by Workers' Compensation, it is probably a good idea to have it. If you are covered, it is debatable (both won't pay): Workers' Compensation will probably take longer to pay for your health care expenses (if you can prove that they are work-related), but it usually pays you for time-off (disability), as well.

Best's Reports *(Is the insuring company any good?)*

If you want to check out an insurance company, your local library should have a copy of Best's Reports that you can use as a reference. A.M. Best Company has been rating, and providing information about insurance companies since 1899, and is the industry's standard. (Standard and Poor's has a similar rating service, but it is focused more on numbers.). Best's rates companies according to financial stability, from as low as "C" to A+ (excellent); but, unlike school grades on a report card, only "As" are acceptable. Ratings of B+ or less, although they don't sound bad, indicate either a shaky or a very young, unproven company.

Best's also provides a history and a listing of corporate officers, along with the company's acitivities and markets. This information is also reproduced in little brochures that are purchased and distributed by the insurance companies and their agents. If an agent doesn't have one, you may want to go to the library. If a company has no rating (not always less than a "C"), it would be worthwhile to find out why.

If you are still leary of a company whose agent (or television commercial) is trying to sell you (solicit) health insurance, you can always ask the BBB (Better Business Bureau) if they have any complaints registered against it. Ask them to also check in the state where the company is domiciled (home office), especially if it is not your home state. Alien (out-of-state) companies can get away with more, but are not necessarily bad, or vice versa. If you don't know the home state of the company (and don't want to, or can't, ask the agent)–it is listed in the Best's Reports.

GLOSSARY
OF SPECIAL TERMS

AHA = American Hospital Association
"Embraced" Blue Cross and helped it prosper.
They saw pre-payment plans as a way of balancing
the books.*

AMA = American Medical Association
(America's largest association of doctors)
They thought that Blue Shield would "socialize"
the fee-for-services relationship of doctor and
patient, by limiting freedom.*

*Rashi Fein's words quoted. (see suggested reading)

Ambulatory Surgical Center
A licensed free-standing facility (or part of a
hospital) solely engaged in providing surgical/
medical servcices on an outpatient basis. You walk
in, and you walk out, on the same day.

Ancillary Services
Operating, delivery and treatment rooms and
equipment; anesthesia supplies and services;
medical and surgical dressings, supplies, casts and
splints; diagnostic and therapeutical services, etc.

Automatic claims filing

Available through some Medicare supplement carriers who automatically receive a copy of the Medicare claim (from Medicare) and pay, accordingly. A good service to have.

Carrier

Generally, an insurer which is usually an insurance company (in health insurance, usually a life insurance company; but, it could be a casualty company). It could be an employer, if the plan is self-insured.

In Medicare = a private insurer contracted to handle claims covered by Part B Medical Insurance.

CMP = Competitive Medical Plan

A prepayment plan like an HMO or even a PPO (preferred provider organization) where you are required to receive health care services directly from their providers, and they are reimbursed (by Medicare) on a monthly "fee-for-service" basis.

Co-insurance, co-payment, cost sharing

The distribution of expenses, by percentage, after the deductible has been satisfied. Most plans are 80% (insurer) and 20% (insured); but, the trend is toward the insured paying a higher percentage, such as 30%, 40% and 50%, on a lower dollar limit. For example: instead of 80/20% on $5,000, it would be 50/50% on $2,000 (or more, later on)...

Complications of pregnancy

1. Conditions (when pregnancy is not ended) whose diagnoses are distinct from pregnancy; but are caused or adversely affected by pregnancy. Some examples: acute nephritis, nephrosis (kidney problems) and cardiac decompensation.

2. Non-elective Caesarian section (usually the first one is covered, the second one is problematic)

3. Ectopic (out of place) pregnancy that is terminated.

4. Spontaneous termination (miscarriage)

5. Missed abortion

Non-complications = False labor, occasional spotting, morning sickness, hyperemis gravidarum, preeclampsia or placenta previa. (Ask your doctor.)

Custodial care

Unskilled treatment or services to help a patient with daily living (survival): walking, bathing, dressing, etc.

Episode

An occurrence (event) of illness or injury, usually in reference to chronic cases when more occurrences are expected.

Full-time student

Usually defined by the school (licensed) that the dependent child is attending. As a general rule, 12 academic hours is probably acceptable; but, it is worth checking with your insurer. (It may be in your policy.)

Hospital

A legally licensed institution whose primary function is to provide medical, diagnostic and surgical facilities, treatment and care for the sick and injured; and is under the direction of a (staff of) doctor (s), and provides 24-hour (graduate) Registered Nursing services (every day).

Individual Practice Association (IPA)

A type of HMO that contracts with private practice physicians for their services on a part-time (discounted) fee-for-service basis.

Inpatient

When you are confined, or stay at least one night in the hospital; be careful of this, if you have special coverage for "outpatient" surgery, etc.

Insurers

Basically, insurance companies who are paid a premium for a policy or certificate (group policy)– not Blue Cross, which has subscribers, or an HMO which has members (they are prepayment plans): The difference seems subtle, but it can be substan- tial if you receive treatment from a non-member provider. PPOs can be a problem in this respect, also. People who travel should be especially concerned. By the way, just because it's "insurance" doesn't mean that it is automatically good anywhere in the world, either. Some policies have stipulations regarding foreign (out-of-the-country) coverage, with time and/or dollar limits. (Read your policy, and check with the company, regarding claims, etc.)

142

Intermediary

Generically, a middle-person or entity that works between the insurer (including self-insured plans) and the insured–one who mediates. In Medicare = someone (usually a company) that handles Part A (hospital) claims.

Managed Medical Systems (MMS)

A combination of an HMO and a PPO which offers the option to use non-member providers; but, under a strict utilization review, and at a cost (out-of-pocket) to you.

Mental illness

Neurosis, phychoneurosis, phychosis, psycho-pathy, or personality disorder.

Morbidity factor

A number (ratio) from a table (like a mortality table in life insurance) that determines the statistical probability of injury and/or illness, by gender and age.

"No gain or no loss" (and vice versa)

When a new (replacing) plan will pay claims on a basis that is neither better or worse than the old plan: If you had a $100 deductible on the old plan, and the new plan has a $250 deductible, it will honor the $100 deductible, and any part of it that has been satisfied (for the first calendar year), so no loss. If you had a $500 deductible on the old plan ($250 on the new), you are stuck with it for a year (or the remainder), so no gain. There are various versions of these plans, so check out the specific language; and, like in the shell game, keep your eye on the pea.

Open enrollment
One time (usually a month) a year when HMOs have to take applicants (so many) regardless (or in spite of) their pre-existing conditions.

Outpatient (same as ambulatory)
Not overnight.

Persistent
The insurance companies' favorite word for business that stays on the books. That is, the premiums keep coming in (on time).

Physician (doctor)
A person (other than you, or a member of your immediate family) who is legally licensed to practice medicine, and qualified to treat the type of illness or injury for which your claim is made, within his/her jurisdiction (state).

Pool adjustment
When all the groups (units) in a trust receive the same (averaged) rate increase (it doesn't usually decrease) regardless of loss experience. It is more in keeping with the idea of health (group) insurance than tier renewal, (further on).

Primary Coverage
In the case of two (or more) prevailing policies (plans), the one that pays first (and usually most). The other(s) may serve as supplemental (secon-

dary) coverage. The decision is usually based on employment (employee vs. spouse) or with individual policies, on longevity (the oldest pays first). Note: Don't expect payment soon. Multiple policies are not a good idea, or recommended.

Stand-Alone
Usually refers to disability, dental or drug plans, when they are purchased separately and not in conjunction with health coverage (especially, from a different carrier).

Third Party Administrator (TPA)
An entity that works as a "middle-man" between insured and insured. Typically a trust, a TPA can be an association (usually for small businesses); they have interesting names, and often go by their initials, such as: N.A.S.E., N.A.C.A., C.B.A. and so forth, and like to use American, National, Consumers, etc., as catchwords. They are not necessarily good or bad—basically, they replace, in a way, people that an insurer would have to hire to handle sales and administrative duties, anyhow.

Tier Renewal
Renewal of premium(s) based on experience: If your group has a high claims/premium ratio, your premium will increase in proportion to it, as you will be categorized with others who have had a similar loss ratio. It's a good question to ask your (prospective) agent. It's not a good situation, if you have a big claim (which is why we have health insurance).

Umbrella coverage

Originally, a kind of major medical policy that covered above and beyond basic hospitalization (Blue Cross). Now, used by self-insurers to cover catastrophic expenses, say $50,000 or more.

Underwriter

A person who works for an insurer, whose job is to decide what risks to accept. This person may accept an applicant, but alter coverage by the use of riders or endorsements that exclude certain pre-existing conditions, or increase the standard premium with a surcharge.

The name comes from when the underwriter(s) would actually sign the contract of insurance (under the writing), like the signers of the Declaration of Independence.

I have a friend who was an underwriter; but, he went into banking, and moved to Philadelphia.

Suggested Reading
(Bibliography)

All About Medicare
The National Underwriter Co., Cincinnati, Ohio. They
publish the "National Underwriter", a monthly
magazine for the insurance industry. They also
publish state versions; for example: "The Ohio
Underwriter." This little book is written in a
question/answer format and goes beyond the free
Medicare brochures. Make sure you get the current annual edition. $5.95 (1989)

The Health Insurance Answer Book
John D. Reynolds and Robin N. Bischoff.
This book is also in a question/answer format; but,
much more technical. It is geared for the medium-
large size employer, or its health insurance person.
It is also expensive for the layperson.
Panel Publishers, $79.95 (1990, 2nd edition).

Source Book of Health Insurance Data
The Health Insurance Institute publishes this
annual informational guide. It contains a little
history; but, is mostly current statistics, graphs, etc.
It is free for members of the Health Insurance
Association of America, and certain libraries
(universities, etc.). This is not a bedside book,
unless you are an accountant or a benefits consult-
ant.

Total Coverage
Darcie Bundy & Stuart Day (spouse)
The authors discuss all types of insurance, with
two chapters on Health Insurance (and a little one
on Disability Income). They seem biased toward
HMOs because of the built-in incentives to control
costs, and the emphasis on preventive care; but,
otherwise a good discussion of HMOs and PPOs.
The Perennial Library (Harper & Row) $10.95 (1987)

Winning the Insurance Game
Ralph Nader & Wesley J. Smith
These two consumer advocate attorneys cover all
types of insurance from auto to Workers' Compensation. I don't particularly agree with some of their
recommendations regarding health insurance,
especially their stance on a National Health Insurance plan; but, they bring up some interesting
points about insurance, in general.
Knight Bridge Publishing Co. $24.95 (1990)

Medical Care, Medical Costs
Rashi Fein
A scholarly (but readable) socio-economic and
political history of health care financing. Dr. Fein
was an advisor on the Medicare Committee and-
presents some interesting insights into the development of Medicare, Medicaid and Health Insurance, in general. He also offers a prescription (a
form of National Health Insurance) for the future.
Harvard University Press. $24.95 (1986)

How to Protect Your Life Savings, from Catastrophic Illness and Nursing Homes
Harley Gordon
This handbook for financial survival of the elderly (and their heirs) is an interesting study written by an attorney, and founding member of the National Academy of Elder Law Attorneys. The author presents a lot of examples and possible scenarios; also, charts of countable assets, allowances, and eligibility standards for Medicaid (by states). *Financial Planning Institute. $18.95 (1990)*

Note: I was able to find the above books either at my local library or the Kent State University Library–and I would like to thank the friendly and helpful people there. Publishers' addresses and phone numbers can be found in the reference section of most libraries.

Avoiding the Medicaid Trap: How to Beat the Catastrophic Costs of Nursing-Home Care
Armond D. Budish
The author, an attorney and prize-winning consumer-law journalist, offers practical strategies and solutions on how to avoid financial devastation from nursing-home costs. This large, (8 1/2 x 11) hardbound book includes power of attorney forms (for all states) and 5 Medicaid trust examples, after a comprehensive discussion of countable assets, eligibility limits, wills, types of ownership, etc., including forms and tables. I even understood most of it–Mom is going to be 79 this year. You might find it in a library. If not, it's $26.95 (postpaid) P.O. Box 24448, Cleveland, OH 44124. *Henry Holt and Company (1990)*

The Complete Guide to Health Insurance
(How to Beat the High Cost of Being Sick)
Kathleen Hogue, Cheryl Jensen and
Kathleen McClurg Wiljanen
Although this book is somewhat outdated in its
treatment of segmented plans (basic coverage
separate from major medical coverage, possibly
through different insurers) and completely outdated in regard to Medicare's Catastrophic coverage (repealed in 1989), the authors give many
examples and strategies (I don't agree with the idea
of having multiple policies, though) in 350+ pages.
Originally in hardcover @ $24.95 (1988), it is now
available (as a large pocketbook) from Avon Books
@ $4.95 + $1.00 handling (call toll-free information
for their 800-number), 1990 printing. It might also
be available at bookstores–I saw it at Walden's.
(The paperback has small print.)

Health Insurance Made Easy...Finally
Sharon L. Stark
For anyone who is interested in, or having problems with, the claims process, this hand/workbook
should help. The author, experienced in claims-
paying, offers this question/fill-in guide with
explanations of specific coverages. It is easy to
read and use, and should save time, and improve
claims returns.
$16.95 (postpaid) 1990 printing–Stark Publishing
P.O. Box 8693 Shawnee Mission, KS 66208.

Index

accident insurance *2*
accident coverage (supplemental) *20-1*
adverse selection (carve-out) *36, 68*
ambulatory surgical center *139*
ancillary services *139*
approved charges *78*
assignment *74-5*
automatic claims filing *140*
Best's Reports *137-8*
birth defects *121*
broker (agent) *51-2*
cafeteria plan *31*
cancer policy *115*
captive agent *51*
carrier *76, 140*
carry-over provision *7, 16*
casualty insurance *1*
check-o-matic (bank draft) *45*
chiropractic care *127*
claims submission *25-6*
COBRA *37-8, 97*
co-insurance (co-payments) *6, 140*
commissions *52*
common accident provision *20*
Competitive Medical Plan (CMP) *140*
complications of pregnancy *141*
Consumer Information Center *80*
contestability period *58-9*
co-ordination of benefits *25*
cosmetic surgery *120*
cost containment *28-9*
custodial care *141*

declinations *132-4*
deductible 15
dependents *122*
Diagnosis-Related Groups (DRG) *75*
episode *141*
exclusions, general *124-5*
exclusions, Medicare *79*
family deductible *20*
full-time student *141*
grace period *45-6*
guaranteed issue *56*
guaranteed renewable *63*
height/weight charts *128-31*
home health care *73, 89*
hospice care *74*
hospital *142*
hospitalization *3*
hospital confinement rider *127*
Individual Practice Association (IPA) *142*
inpatient *142*
insurer *142*
interim insurance *135-6*
intermediary *76, 143*
late entry, applicant *67-8*
major medical *5, 49*
Managed Medical System (MMS) *143*
marital counseling *123*
Medical Information Bureau *64, 136*
mental illness *125-6, 143*
morbidity factor *143*
Multiple Employer Trust (MET) *50*
no gain or no loss *47, 143-4*
non-renewing clause *66*
OBRA *38*
open enrollment *62, 144*

overcharges *17-8*
out-of-pocket expense *6, 16*
outpatient surgery *24, 144*
Peer Review Organization (PRO) *75*
per cause plan *7*
permanent rider *58*
physician (doctor) *144*
physiotherapy *125-6*
pool adjustment *144*
prescriptions *34-5*
primary coverage *144-5*
Prospective Payment Systems (PPS) *75*
psychiatric care *125-6*
Quality Review Organization (QRO) *77*
quick-pay *40*
second-opinion surgery *119*
skilled nursing facility (SNF) *72*
stand-alone plan *145*
step-rate *43-4*
surcharge *131-2*
temporomandibular joint (TMJ) *120*
third party administrator (TPA) *145*
tier renewal *145*
transplant surgery *133*
trend (inflation) *54*
twenty-four hour coverage *137*
umbrella coverage *146*
underwriter *146*
utilization review *28-9*
weight loss surgery *120*

Instructions
How to get the most from this book

First, read the book through at your leisure.

Second, find your health insurance policy.

Third, read the policy and try to imagine some of the possible scenarios that you could get into, and how the policy would cover them.

Fourth, discuss health insurance with friends and/or fellow workers. Depending on the situation, you may be able to discuss specific episodes and their consequences of coverage.

Fifth, after a time, and some experience (real, imagined, or second-hand), read the book again.

Sixth, repeat second through fifth steps....